POCKET GUIDE TO
PSYCHIATRIC PRACTICE

A Companion to the Introductory
Textbook of Psychiatry, Sixth Edition

POCKET GUIDE TO
PSYCHIATRIC PRACTICE

A Companion to the Introductory
Textbook of Psychiatry, Sixth Edition

Donald W. Black, M.D.

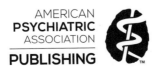

AMERICAN
PSYCHIATRIC
ASSOCIATION
PUBLISHING

Copyright © 2018 American Psychiatric Association

ALL RIGHTS RESERVED

First Edition

Manufactured in the United States of America on acid-free paper
22   21   20   19   18   5   4   3   2   1

American Psychiatric Association Publishing
800 Maine Ave., SW, Suite 900
Washington, DC 20024-2812
www.appi.org

Library of Congress Cataloging-in-Publication Data
Names: Black, Donald W., author. | Supplement to (expression): Black, Donald W., Introductory textbook of psychiatry. Sixth edition. | American Psychiatric Association, issuing body.
Title: Pocket guide to psychiatric practice / Donald W. Black.
Description: First edition. | Washington, DC : American Psychiatric Association Publishing, [2018] | Companion to Introductory textbook of psychiatry / Donald W. Black. Sixth edition. [2014]. | Includes bibliographical references and index.
Identifiers: LCCN 2018005038 (print) | LCCN 2018005529 (ebook) | ISBN 9781615371983 (ebook) | ISBN 9781615371549 (pbk. : alk.   paper)
Subjects: | MESH: Mental Disorders—diagnosis | Mental Disorders—therapy | Psychiatry | Handbooks
Classification: LCC RC454.4 (ebook) | LCC RC454.4 (print) | NLM WM 34 | DDC 616.89—dc23
LC record available at https://lccn.loc.gov/2018005038

British Library Cataloguing in Publication Data
A CIP record is available from the British Library.

Contents

PART III
SPECIAL TOPICS

About the Author

Donald W. Black, M.D., is Professor of Psychiatry at the University of Iowa Roy J. and Lucille A. Carver College of Medicine in Iowa City, Iowa. He is a graduate of Stanford University, where he received his undergraduate degree, and the University of Utah School of Medicine. He received his psychiatric training at the University of Iowa Hospitals and Clinics and completed a fellowship in psychiatric epidemiology. Dr. Black serves as Director of Residency Training and Vice Chair for Education in the Department of Psychiatry. He has authored or coauthored several books, including *Bad Boys, Bad Men: Confronting Antisocial Personality Disorder (Sociopathy)* and *DSM-5® Guidebook*. He is a Distinguished Fellow of the American Psychiatric Association and is past President of the American Academy of Clinical Psychiatrists.

The author has no competing interests to report.

Preface

This pocket guide to psychiatric practice, a companion to *Introductory Textbook of Psychiatry*, now in its sixth edition ("DSM-5 version"), was prompted by requests from medical students and residents for a more user-friendly version of the textbook that they could easily carry with them. Although many students and residents no longer wear white lab coats with generous pockets that we traditionally associate with the practice of medicine, this version is portable and concise. Yet it continues the tradition Nancy Andreasen and I started in 1991. Our goal was to write a highly readable, interesting, and useful text to guide learners as they begin their journey in psychiatry. Using this book as a tool, students will learn to enjoy working with psychiatric patients of all types and in all settings.

As Nancy and I observed, psychiatry is the most human of the medical specialties, and all learners—regardless of what they do in the future—should be able to define and recognize mental illnesses, to identify methods for treating them, and, for those few who become researchers, to help develop methods for discovering their causes and implementing preventive measures.

This pocket guide is compatible with DSM-5, the fifth edition of *Diagnostic and Statistical Manual of Mental Disorders*. The text is organized, as in DSM-5, to follow the developmental lifespan and includes DSM-5 criteria sets (with codes and, in most cases, specifiers and subtypes left out for purposes of the pocket guide format) for the most common disorders that learners encounter.

Pocket Guide to Psychiatric Practice is a companion to the larger and more detailed *Introductory Textbook of Psychiatry*, as well as to *Study Guide to Introductory Psychiatry*. For those dedicated to learning the ins and outs of psychiatric disorders and their assessment, these books set the stage for lifelong learning. The book also joins the family of publications from American Psychiatric Association Publishing that have become vital teaching resources.

Although the book is written primarily for medical students and residents in their first years of training, it will be useful for individuals seeking psychiatric training from the perspectives of other disciplines, such as nursing or social work.

I wish to thank the many students, residents, and colleagues who have provided important feedback over the years. Special thanks go to Nancy Andreasen, who has been a valued friend and mentor and was instrumental for encouraging me—then a very junior faculty member—to join her in writing the first edition of *Introductory Textbook of Psychiatry*. Little did I realize that the book would thrive throughout its now six editions, be translated into six languages, and achieve worldwide distribution.

I wish to thank the talented staff at American Psychiatric Association Publishing—including Editor-in-Chief Laura Roberts and Interim Publisher John McDuffie, who provided needed encouragement and support—who have made this book possible.

Last, although this guide has been reviewed many times, it is possible that there are inadvertent errors. Please feel free to contact the author at donald-black@uiowa.edu with your thoughts or comments.

PART I

Diagnosis and Psychiatric Interview

Chapter 1

Diagnosis and Classification

Creating order out of chaos and improving physician-to-physician communication are some of the many goals of diagnosis. To facilitate this process, in the United States psychiatric diagnoses are based on the *Diagnostic and Statistical Manual of Mental Disorders* (DSM), now in its fifth edition (DSM-5). Outside of the United States, diagnosis likely is based on the World Health Organization's (WHO's) *International Classification of Diseases* (ICD), now in its tenth revision (ICD-10).

Why Diagnose Patients?

Main Purposes of Diagnoses

- **Diagnoses introduce order and structure to our thinking and reduce the complexity of clinical phenomena.** Disorders are divided into broad classes based on common features, creating a structure within the apparent chaos of clinical phenomena that makes mental illnesses easier to learn about and understand.
- **Diagnoses facilitate communication among clinicians.** The use of diagnostic categories gives clinicians a kind of "shorthand" through which they can summarize large quantities of information relatively easily.
- **Diagnoses help to predict outcome.** Many psychiatric diagnoses are associated with a characteristic course and outcome. Bipolar I disorder, for example, usually is episodic, with periods of "highs" and "lows," and has a relatively good outcome with treatment.
- **Diagnoses often are used to choose an appropriate treatment.** Relatively specific treatments for particular disorders or groups of symptoms have been developed. For example, antipsychotic drugs typically are used to treat psy-

choses. A diagnosis of mania suggests the use of a mood stabilizer such as lithium carbonate or valproate.

- **Diagnoses can help guide research on pathophysiology and etiology.** Knowledge about specific groupings of clinical symptoms might correlate with information about brain specialization and function so that hypotheses about the neurochemical or anatomical basis of a particular disorder can be formulated.

Other Purposes of Diagnoses

- **Diagnoses are used to monitor treatment and to make decisions about reimbursement.** As health care has become more managed, diagnoses often are used to determine the length of a hospital stay or the choice of a treatment course for a specific condition.
- **Diagnoses are used by attorneys in malpractice suits and other litigation.** As DSM has made the diagnostic system of psychiatry more open and accessible, lawyers and patients have learned much more about psychiatric classification.
- **Diagnoses are used by health care epidemiologists to determine the incidence and prevalence of various diseases throughout the world.** Diagnoses recorded in hospital or clinic charts are used to track regional differences in disease patterns as well as changes over time.

The Story Behind DSM

The impetus to organize DSM began during World War II. Shortly thereafter, the American Psychiatric Association convened a committee to develop a diagnostic manual. The first DSM (referred to as DSM-I) was published in 1952. Over the years, the DSM has undergone four major revisions (DSM-II, DSM-III, DSM-IV, and DSM-5). Currently, as noted earlier, psychiatric diagnoses are based on DSM-5, published in 2013.

The early handbooks were relatively short. DSM-I had 132 pages and DSM-II contained 119 pages (excluding front matter). DSM-III, which was released in 1980, was the first effort by a medical specialty to provide a comprehensive and detailed diagnostic manual in which all disorders were defined by specific criteria.

DSM-III, at 494 pages, was considered transformative. By introducing criteria, the process of diagnosis was greatly simplified and helped change the way psychiatrists and other mental health professionals engage in the diagnostic process. Research investigations showed that different clinicians using DSM-I or DSM-II guidelines gave different diagnoses to the same patient. The authors of DSM-III created diagnostic criteria that were as objective as possible, and they based their decisions on available research data whenever possible. They largely achieved this goal and helped to change what had been an often arbitrary practice of psychiatric diagnosis. DSM-IV and DSM-5 continued the practice of including objective and reliable diagnostic criteria.

Advantages and Disadvantages of DSM

Advantages

- **The DSM system has substantially improved reliability of diagnosis.** *Reliability*, a biometric concept, refers to the ability of two observers to agree on what they see. The reliability of psychiatric diagnosis ranges from good to excellent for most major categories.
- **The DSM system has clarified the diagnostic process and facilitated history taking.** DSM-5 is highly objective because it specifies which symptoms must be present to make a diagnosis. The DSM system brings signs and symptoms to the forefront of evaluation.
- **The DSM system has clarified and facilitated the process of differential diagnosis.** DSM helps clinicians decide which symptoms must be present to rule in or to rule out a specific diagnosis. For example, it specifies that a schizophrenia diagnosis cannot be made if mood episodes have been present for a majority of the total duration of the illness.

Disadvantages

- **The increased precision sometimes gives clinicians and researchers a false sense of certainty about what they are doing.** Although diagnostic criteria are based on data whenever possible, the available research often is inadequate or incomplete, and this makes the selection of signs and symptoms arbitrary at times. The diagnoses themselves are certainly arbitrary and will remain so as long as we are ignorant about pathophysiology and etiology.

- **The DSM system might sacrifice validity for reliability.** *Reliability* refers to the capacity of individuals to agree on what they see, whereas *validity* refers to the ability to predict prognosis and outcome, response to treatment, and ultimately etiology. Therefore, the question remains: although a disorder could be reliable, is it valid?
- **The DSM system could encourage clinicians to treat diagnosis as a checklist and forget about the patient as a person.** DSM-5 can be used to streamline clinical interviews because it encourages the use of a checklist of symptoms. There is nothing wrong with the checklist approach, but its use can interfere with establishing a close doctor–patient relationship and learning about the patient's life and relationships.

Learning to Use DSM-5

DSM-5 is large (947 pages, excluding front matter) and complex. Rather than attempt to master everything at once, clinicians in training should focus on the major classes and categories seen in psychiatric practice or in primary care settings, such as schizophrenia, major depression, or substance use disorders. DSM-5 begins with the neurodevelopmental disorders, often diagnosed in infancy and early childhood, and progresses through diagnostic areas more commonly diagnosed in adulthood, such as sleep-wake disorders. Table 1–1 lists the major diagnostic classes in DSM-5.

Recording a Diagnosis

After a clinician has completed the data-gathering process (described in the next chapter), diagnostic possibilities should be rank ordered, and diagnoses that are unlikely should be discarded or ruled out. This is the process of *differential diagnosis*. It is not unusual for the diagnostic process to continue as additional information is gathered. With few exceptions, DSM-5 encourages clinicians to make several diagnoses when necessary to fully describe the patient's condition.

TABLE 1–1. DSM-5 diagnostic categories

Neurodevelopmental disorders

Schizophrenia spectrum and other psychotic disorders

Bipolar and related disorders

Depressive disorders

Anxiety disorders

Obsessive-compulsive and related disorders

Trauma- and stressor-related disorders

Dissociative disorders

Somatic symptom and related disorders

Feeding and eating disorders

Elimination disorders

Sleep-wake disorders

Sexual dysfunctions

Gender dysphoria

Disruptive, impulse-control, and conduct disorders

Substance-related and addictive disorders

Neurocognitive disorders

Personality disorders

Paraphilic disorders

Other mental disorders

Diagnoses are ranked in order of their focus of attention or treatment, with the condition primarily responsible for a patient's hospital stay (or outpatient visit) listed as the *principal diagnosis* (or *reason for visit*), which may be written parenthetically after the diagnosis—for example, "(principal diagnosis)." The exception is when the mental disorder is caused by a medical condition, in which case *that* medical condition is listed first. For example, if an outpatient with HIV seeks care for symptoms related to a mild neurocognitive disorder caused by the HIV, "HIV infection" is listed first, followed by "mild neurocognitive disorder due to HIV infection (reason for visit)."

If there is insufficient information to establish a firm diagnosis and there is a strong presumption that the diagnosis will be met, the clinician could indicate this uncertainty by recording "(provisional)" after the diagnosis.

Sometimes it is difficult to determine the patient's principal diagnosis or reason for visit, particularly when multiple conditions are present (e.g., is the patient's schizophrenia or alcohol use disorder the main problem?). Any diagnostic list will appear arbitrary to a certain extent, and although we all crave certainty, it might not be possible.

Two examples illustrate how a clinician might record a diagnosis (or diagnoses) after an evaluation:

Example 1

A 25-year-old man is brought to the emergency room by family members for bizarre behavior, including making threats of harm, muttering obscenities, and talking to himself. His bizarre behavior appears motivated by paranoid delusions. Family members report that he drinks nearly daily to intoxication and smokes cigarettes almost nonstop. He has had several prior hospitalizations for similar features and has been diagnosed with schizophrenia. His DSM-5 diagnoses are:

- Schizophrenia (principal diagnosis)
- Alcohol use disorder, moderate
- Tobacco use disorder, severe

Example 2

A 65-year-old man is brought to the clinic by his worried wife. She reports that he has been diagnosed with lung cancer, which his doctors believe has metastasized to his brain. He hears "voices" that tell him not to trust family members. He has become very suspicious and has threatened family members who he believes are planning to kill him. He has no psychiatric history. His DSM-5 diagnoses are:

- Malignant lung neoplasm
- Psychosis due to malignant lung neoplasm (provisional)

DSM-5 does *not* include treatment guidelines. Nonetheless, accurate diagnosis is the first step in providing appropriate treatment for any medical condition, and mental disorders are no exception. Despite the absence of treatment information,

TABLE 1–2. Clinically useful information in DSM-5 for each diagnosis

Subtypes and/or specifiers (where applicable)

Recording procedures (where applicable)

Diagnostic features

Associated features supporting diagnosis

Prevalence

Development and course

Risk and prognostic factors

Culture-related diagnostic issues

Gender-related diagnostic issues

Diagnostic markers

Suicide risk

Functional consequences

Differential diagnosis

Comorbidity

DSM-5 provides a wealth of information about diagnostic classification and disorders that learners of all backgrounds will find useful. These resources are detailed in Table 1–2.

DSM-5 Coding and ICD

The official diagnostic coding system in the United States is not DSM-5 but the *International Classification of Diseases, Tenth Revision, Clinical Modification* (ICD-10-CM), originally released by WHO in 2010, with codes taking effect in October 2015. The ICD is a global classification system created more than 100 years ago and includes all medical and mental health conditions.

The word *code* refers to the 3- to 5-digit number that follows the name of the disorder and accompanies the criteria set. Some disorders have *subtypes* and *specifiers* that provide increased diagnostic specificity. Subtypes are mutually exclusive and specifiers are not.

Further Reading

American Psychiatric Association: Diagnostic and Statistical Manual of Mental Disorders, 5th Edition. Arlington, VA, American Psychiatric Association, 2013

Black DW, Grant JE: DSM-5 Guidebook: The Essential Companion to the Diagnostic and Statistical Manual of Mental Disorders, 5th Edition. Washington, DC, American Psychiatric Publishing, 2014

Decker H: The Making of DSM-III: A Diagnostic Manual's Conquest of American Psychiatry. New York, Oxford University Press, 2013

Wilson M: DSM-III and the transformation of American psychiatry: a history. Am J Psychiatry 150(3):399–410, 1993

Chapter 2

Interviewing and Assessment

The Psychiatric Interview

An initial psychiatric interview serves the following purposes:

- To formulate an impression of the patient's diagnosis or differential diagnosis and to begin to generate a treatment plan
- To produce a document that contains information organized in a standard, readable, and easily interpretable way
- To help the clinician establish a therapeutic relationship with the patient and reassure him or her that help will be provided

A standard psychiatric interview is similar to standard interviews conducted in the rest of medicine, with some minor modifications. The content of the present illness and patient history is focused primarily on psychiatric symptoms, while the family history includes more detailed information about psychiatric illnesses among family members. Social history also includes more personal information than is recorded in the standard medical history. An important part of the interview—the mental status examination (MSE)—is the psychiatrist's equivalent to an internist's physical examination. The psychiatric evaluation is outlined in Table 2–1.

Identification of the Patient and Informants

Identify the patient by age, race, gender, partnered status, and occupation. Is the patient the sole informant, or has collateral history been obtained (from prior records, family members, or others)? Indicate if the patient is self-referred, has been brought in at the request of family members, or has been referred by a physician. Is the patient a reliable historian?

TABLE 2–1. Elements of the psychiatric evaluation

Identification of the patient and informants

Chief complaint

History of present illness

Psychiatric history

Family history

Social history

General medical history

Mental status examination

General physical examination and neurological examination

Diagnostic impression

Treatment and management plan

Chief Complaint

Use the patient's own words (e.g., "I'm thinking of killing myself," or "The voices tell me to hurt people"). An additional sentence or two of additional information may be provided, particularly if the patient's chief complaint is vague.

History of Present Illness

Provide a concise history of the illness or problem that brought the patient to the hospital or clinic. Describe symptom onset. If this is the patient's first episode, psychiatric evaluation, or hospital admission, state this early in the history of the present illness. Indicate when the first symptoms began, the nature of onset (e.g., acute, insidious), and whether onset was precipitated by any specific life events or problems. Identify medical conditions that could be causing significant stress. Note if drug or alcohol abuse is a problem or stressor.

Describe the evolution of the patient's symptoms. This listing of symptoms should reflect DSM-5 criteria and should specify which symptoms are present and which are absent. The description should not be limited to symptoms included in the diagnostic criteria, however, because these criteria typically do not provide a full description of the range of symptoms that patients experience. The description of the present illness also should indicate the degree of distress and disability that the patient is experiencing. Record any medications the patient has taken for the present illness, including dosages, duration, and effectiveness.

Psychiatric History

This portion of the history will be extensive if the patient has a long and complex illness. Begin by noting the patient's age when he or she was first seen for psychiatric evaluation and the number of hospitalizations or episodes. Thereafter, describe past episodes in chronological order, with information about duration of episodes, types of symptoms present, severity of symptoms, treatments received, and response to treatment.

Family History

Note the age and occupation of parents, siblings, and children (if applicable). If any first-degree relatives (parents, siblings, children) have a history of any mental illness, list the specific illness, along with information about treatment, hospitalization, and long-term course and outcome. Obtain as much information as possible about mental illness in the extended family as well. Draw pedigrees in complicated cases.

Social History

The social history captures more than if the patient smokes, drinks, or uses drugs. This section should provide a concise report of the patient's life story: where the patient was born and raised; the nature of early life adjustment; problems during childhood, such as temper tantrums, school phobia, or delinquency; relationships with parents and siblings; and sexual development. Include information about the patient's religious or cultural attitudes, educational history, interests and participation in extracurricular activities, and interpersonal relationships. Summarize work history and military history.

Detail the patient's current social situation, including marital (or partnered) status, occupation, and income. Note if the patient is disabled. Describe the location of the patient's residence, as well as the specific family members who live with the patient. This section of the history should provide information about social supports currently available to the patient. Record use of tobacco, alcohol, and illicit drugs.

General Medical History

Note any existing medical illness for which the patient is currently receiving treatment, as well as the types of treatments, medications, and their dosages. Include vitamins, supplements, herbals, or other alternative or complementary treatments (e.g., acupuncture, chiropractic care, homeopathy). Summarize allergies, past surgeries, traumatic injuries, or other serious medical illnesses. Head injuries, headaches, seizures, and other problems involving the CNS are particularly relevant.

Mental Status Examination

The MSE assesses the patient's appearance, critical thinking, speech patterns, memory, and judgment. Some domains are determined simply by observing the patient (e.g., appearance, affect). Other portions are elucidated by asking relatively specific questions (e.g., mood, abnormalities in perception). Still others are assessed by asking the patient a specified set of questions (e.g., memory, general information).

The interviewer should develop his or her own approach to assessing mental functions such as memory, general information, and calculation, which should be used consistently for all patients so that the clinician develops a sense of the range of normal and abnormal responses. Components of the MSE are summarized in Table 2–2.

Appearance and Attitude

Describe the patient's general appearance. Does the patient look older than his or her stated age? Note the patient's grooming/hygiene and appropriateness of dress. Describe the patient's attitude toward the interview (cooperative, guarded, angry, or suspicious).

Motor Activity

Record the patient's level of motor activity. Does the patient sit quietly, or is he or she physically agitated? Note any abnormal movements, tics, or mannerisms. Is there evidence of catatonia (waxy flexibility, rigidity, or mutism)?

TABLE 2–2. Features of the mental status examination

Appearance and attitude	General information
Motor activity	Calculations
Thought and speech	Capacity to read and write
Mood and affect	Visuospatial ability
Perception	Attention
Orientation	Abstraction
Memory	Judgment and insight

Thought and Speech

Note the patient's pattern and rate of speech. Is speech logical and goal directed (linear), or is it disordered or even incoherent? If the latter, the patient can be described as having a *formal thought disorder*. Summarize the content of thought, noting any delusional thinking that is present.

Mood and Affect

Describe the patient's mood and affect. The term *mood* refers to an emotional attitude that is relatively sustained and usually is determined by the patient's self-report. Note whether the patient's mood is neutral, euphoric, depressed, anxious, or irritable. *Affect* refers to the way a patient conveys his or her emotional state, as perceived by others. Affect typically is described as full, flat, blunted, or inappropriate. *Flat* or *blunted affect* is inferred when the patient shows little emotional response and seems emotionally dulled. *Inappropriate affect* refers to emotional responses that are not appropriate (e.g., silly laughter when asked about something sad).

Perception

Record any perceptual abnormalities. The most common are *hallucinations*: abnormal sensory perceptions in the absence of an actual stimulus. Hallucinations can be auditory, visual, tactile, or olfactory. An *illusion* is a misinterpretation of an actual stimulus (e.g., seeing a shadow and believing it is a man).

Orientation

Ask the patient to describe the day, date, year, time, place where he or she is currently residing, his or her name and identity, and why he or she is in the hospital (or clinic).

Memory

Memory is divided into very short term, short term, and long term. *Very-short-term memory* involves the immediate registration of information, typically assessed by asking the patient to immediately repeat a series of digits or three pieces of information (e.g., orange, airplane, tobacco). If the patient has difficulty, give him or her the items repeatedly until he or she is able to register them. If the patient is unable to register them after three or four trials, this should be noted. Then tell the patient that he or she will be asked to recall these items in 3 to 5 minutes. The ability to remember these items after that time interval is an indication of *short-term memory*. *Long-term memory* is assessed by asking the patient to recall events that occurred in the last several days, as well as events that occurred in the more remote past, such as months or years ago.

General Information

Ask the patient a set of questions covering topics such as the names of the last five presidents, current events, or information about history or geography. Note the patient's fund of general information in relation to his or her level of educational achievement.

Calculations

The standard test of calculations is serial 7s. This test involves having the patient subtract 7 from 100, then 7 from that difference, and so on for at least five subtractions. Poorly educated patients may need to calculate serial 3s. Likewise, real-life calculations can be simplified or made more complex (e.g., "If I went to the store and bought six oranges, priced at three for a dollar, and gave the clerk a $10 bill, how much change would I get back?").

Capacity to Read and Write

Give the patient a simple text and ask him or her to read it aloud. The patient also should be asked to write down a specific sentence, either of the examiner's choice or of the patient's choice. Assess the patient's ability to read and write relative to his or her educational level.

Visuospatial Ability

Ask the patient to copy a figure. This figure can be quite simple, such as a square inside a circle. An alternative task is to ask the patient to draw a clock face and set the hands at a specified time, such as 10 minutes past 11 o'clock.

Attention

Attention is assessed in part by using calculations or clock setting. Additional tests of attention can be used, such as asking the patient to spell a word backward (e.g., "world"). The patient also can be asked to name five things that start with a specific letter, such as *d*.

Abstraction

The patient's capacity to think abstractly can be assessed in a variety of ways. One method is to ask the patient to interpret a proverb, such as "The tongue is the enemy of the neck." Or, the patient can be asked to identify similarities between two items (e.g., "How are an apple and an orange alike?").

Judgment and Insight

Assess overall judgment and insight by noting how realistically the patient has appraised his or her illness. The clinician can ask: "Do you believe you are mentally ill?" or "Do you believe you need treatment?" Judgment might not be as easily assessed, but the patient's recent choices and decisions will help in its determination. Sometimes simple questions can help (e.g., "If you found a stamped, addressed envelope, what would you do?").

Many psychiatrists routinely administer quick paper-and-pencil tests to assess mental status, most commonly the Mini Mental State Examination (MMSE). An alternative to the MMSE is the Montreal Cognitive Assessment (MoCA). Both assess multiple cognitive domains.

General Physical Examination

The physical examination should follow the standard format used in the rest of medicine, covering organ systems from head to foot. Examinations of patients of the opposite sex (e.g., male physician examining a female patient) should be chaperoned. Include a standard neurological examination.

Diagnostic Impression

List all DSM-5 diagnoses for which the patient's symptoms meet diagnostic criteria. Rank order diagnoses in terms of importance or relevance to the situation.

Treatment and Management Plan

The first step might be to seek additional laboratory tests, brain imaging, or neuropsychological tests (e.g., tests of attention, memory, and cognition) that can assist in the differential diagnosis. If the diagnosis is straightforward, a treatment plan can be outlined, including proposed medication, referral for psychosocial treatments, couples counseling, or other appropriate treatments.

Interviewing Methods

- **Establish rapport early in the interview.** The overall tone of the opening of the interview should convey warmth and friendliness. Once rapport has been established, the interviewer should focus on the patient's problems that led him or her to seek care. Do not allow modern technology (e.g., electronic medical records) to interfere with rapport. The patient is more important than a desktop computer!
- **Determine the chief complaint.** The initial portion of the interview, devoted to eliciting the chief complaint, should take as long as is necessary to determine the patient's primary problem. If the patient is a poor historian, the clinician will need to be active and directive.
- **Use the chief complaint to develop a provisional differential diagnosis.** Once the patient's primary problem has been determined, begin to construct a list of possible diagnoses. For example, if the patient hears voices, possibilities include schizophrenia, schizoaffective disorder, a psychotic mood disorder, or a drug-induced psychosis.
- **Rule out or in the various diagnostic possibilities by using more focused and detailed questions.** If the patient's chief complaint suggests three or four possible diagnoses,

determine which is most relevant by referring to the diagnostic criteria of those disorders.

- **Follow up vague or obscure replies with enough persistence to accurately determine the answer to the question.** Some patients, specifically psychotic patients, have great difficulty answering questions clearly and concisely. They might say "yes" or "no" to every question asked. When this type of pattern is observed, repeatedly ask the patient to describe his or her experiences as explicitly as possible.
- **Let the patient talk freely enough to observe how tightly his or her thoughts are connected.** Most patients should be allowed to talk for at least 3 or 4 minutes without interruption during any psychiatric interview. The coherence of the pattern of the patient's thoughts as presented could provide major clues to the type of problem that he or she is experiencing.
- **Use a mixture of open and closed questions.** Interviewers can learn a great deal about patients by mixing up their types of questions. Open-ended questions permit the patient to ramble and become disorganized, whereas closed questions determine whether the patient can come up with specifics when pressed.
- **Do not be afraid to ask about topics that you or the patient might find difficult or embarrassing.** Beginning interviewers might find it difficult to ask about sexual relationships, sexual experiences, or even use of alcohol or drugs. Yet this information is part of a complete psychiatric interview and must be included. Nearly all patients expect doctors to ask these questions and are not offended.
- **Do not forget to ask about suicidal thoughts.** This subject can be broached tactfully by a question such as "Have you ever felt life isn't worth living?" The topic of suicide can then be discussed, leading to more specific questions (see Chapter 18 for sample questions).
- **Give the patient a chance to ask questions at the end.** Ask a patient, "Is there anything you feel is important that we haven't talked about?" Even if the patient's responses are not helpful to the diagnostic process, they are significant to the patient and therefore intrinsically important.
- **Conclude the initial interview by conveying a sense of confidence and, if possible, hope.** Thank the patient for providing so much information. Compliment him or her on having told his or her story well. Indicate that you now have

a much better understanding of his or her problems, and conclude by stating that you will do what you can to help.

Common Signs and Symptoms and Methods for Eliciting Them

Psychotic Symptoms

Psychotic symptoms involve impairment in the ability to make judgments about the boundaries between what is real and not real (sometimes called "impaired reality testing"). At a more operational level, psychosis is synonymous with having delusions and hallucinations. A somewhat broader definition also includes bizarre behavior, disorganized speech ("positive formal thought disorder"), and inappropriate affect, also known as *positive symptoms*. A second group of symptoms, referred to as *negative symptoms*, occur primarily in schizophrenia and include alogia, affective blunting, avolition–apathy, anhedonia–asociality, and attentional impairment.

Delusions

Delusions are fixed false beliefs that cannot be explained by the patient's cultural background. Assessment should take into account their persistence, their complexity, whether the patient acts on them, the extent to which the patient doubts them, and the degree to which the beliefs deviate from those of nonpsychotic people. Beliefs held with less than a delusional intensity are called *overvalued ideas*.

Persecutory delusions. The patient believes that he or she is being conspired against or persecuted in some way.

- Have you felt that people are against you?
- Has anyone been trying to harm you in any way?

Delusions of jealousy. The patient believes that his or her spouse or partner is having an affair.

- Are you worried that your (husband, wife, boyfriend, girlfriend) might be unfaithful to you?

Delusions of sin or guilt. The patient believes that he or she has committed some terrible sin or done something unforgivable.

- Have you felt that you have done some terrible thing?
- Is there anything that is bothering your conscience?

Grandiose delusions.   The patient believes that he or she has special powers or abilities, is a famous person, has written a definitive book, or has created an amazing invention.

- Do you have any special powers, talents, or abilities?
- Do you feel you are going to achieve great things?

Religious delusions.   The patient is preoccupied with false beliefs of a religious nature. The patient might believe he or she is the Messiah or is leading a new religious movement.

- Have you had any unusual religious experiences?
- Have you become closer to God?

Somatic delusions.   The patient believes that somehow his or her body is diseased, abnormal, or changed. For example, the patient might believe that his or her stomach or brain is rotting.

- Is there anything wrong with the way your body is working?
- Have you noticed any change in your appearance?

Delusions of reference.   The patient believes that insignificant remarks, statements, or events have some special meaning for him or her. For example, the patient walks into a room, sees people laughing, and suspects that they were talking about him or her.

- Have you walked into a room and thought that people were talking about you or laughing at you?
- Have you seen things in magazines, on TV, or on your computer that seem to refer to you or contain a special message meant for you?

Delusions of passivity (being controlled).   The patient has a subjective experience that his or her feelings or actions are controlled by an outside force—for example, that his or her body has been occupied by an alien force that is making it move in peculiar ways, or that messages are being sent to his or her brain by radio waves.

- Have you felt that you were being controlled by some outside person or force?
- Do you sometimes feel like a puppet on a string?

Delusions of mind reading.   The patient believes people can read his or her mind or know his or her thoughts.

- Have you had the feeling that people can read your mind or know what you are thinking?

Thought broadcasting and audible thoughts.   The patient believes that his or her thoughts are broadcast so that he or she or others can hear them. Sometimes the patient believes that his or her thoughts are picked up by a microphone and broadcast on the radio, television, or through the Internet.

- Have you heard your own thoughts out loud, as if they were a voice outside your head?
- Have you felt that your thoughts were broadcast so that other people could hear them?

Thought insertion.   The patient believes that thoughts that are not the patient's own have been inserted into his or her mind.

- Have you felt that thoughts were being placed into your head by some outside person or force?

Thought withdrawal.   The patient believes that thoughts have been taken away from his or her mind.

- Have you felt that your thoughts were taken away by some outside person or force?

Hallucinations

Hallucinations are false perceptions that are occurring in the absence of an identifiable external stimulus and that might be experienced in any of the sensory modalities, including hearing, touch, taste, smell, and vision.

Auditory hallucinations.   Auditory hallucinations typically involve hearing voices speaking to the patient or calling his or her name. The voices could be male or female, familiar or unfamiliar, or critical or complimentary. Hallucinations involving sounds other than voices are less characteristic.

- Have you heard voices or other sounds when no one was around or when you could not account for them?

Voices commenting.   These hallucinations involve hearing a voice that makes a running commentary on the patient's behavior as it occurs (e.g., "Carl is brushing his teeth").

- Have you heard voices commenting on what you are thinking or doing?

Voices conversing.   These hallucinations involve hearing two or more voices talking with each other.

- Have you heard two or more voices talking with one another?

Somatic or tactile hallucinations.   These hallucinations involve experiencing peculiar physical sensations in the body, such as burning, itching, or tingling sensations.

- Have you had burning sensations or other strange sensations in your body?

Olfactory hallucinations.   The patient experiences unusual odors that typically are quite unpleasant. Sometimes the patient reports that he or she smells bad.

- Have you experienced any unusual smells or smells that others do not notice?

Visual hallucinations.   The patient sees shapes or people that are not actually present.

- Have you had visions or seen things that other people cannot?

Bizarre or Disorganized Behavior

The patient's behavior is unusual, bizarre, or fantastic.

Clothing and appearance.   The patient dresses in an unusual manner or does other strange things to alter his or her appearance. The patient's clothing could be inappropriate to the climatic conditions, such as heavy wools in summer.

- Has anyone made comments about the way you dress or appear?

Social behavior.   The patient might do things that are considered inappropriate according to usual social norms. For example, he or she may urinate or defecate in public, or walk along the street muttering to himself or herself.

- Have you done anything that others might think is unusual or that has called attention to yourself?
- Has anyone complained or commented about your behavior?

Aggressive and agitated behavior.   The patient might behave in an aggressive, agitated manner, often quite unpredictably.

- Have you been unusually angry or irritable with anyone?
- Have you done anything to try to harm animals or people?

Ritualistic or stereotyped behavior.   The patient may develop a set of repetitive actions or rituals that he or she must perform over and over. Sometimes the patient will attribute symbolic significance to these actions and believe that they are either influencing others or preventing himself or herself from being influenced.

- Are there any things that you do over and over?
- Are there any things that you have to do in a certain way or in a particular order?

Disorganized Speech
(Positive Formal Thought Disorder)

Disorganized speech is fluent speech that tends to communicate poorly. The patient might skip from topic to topic without warning, or is distracted by events in the environment. He or she might join words together because they are semantically or phonologically alike, even though they make no sense; or ignore the question asked and answer another. To evaluate for thought disorder, allow the patient to talk without interruption for as long as 5 minutes and listen closely. See Table 2–3 for types of disorganized speech (formal thought disorder).

TABLE 2–3. Types of disorganized speech (formal thought disorder)

Derailment (loose associations)	Spontaneous speech in which ideas slip off track and onto another that is obliquely related or unrelated. The speech comes across as disjointed.
Tangentiality	Responding to a question in a tangential or irrelevant manner.
Incoherence	Speech that is incomprehensible, involving unclear or confusing connections between thoughts.
Illogicality	A speaking style in which illogical conclusions are reached. Illogicality can take the form of non sequiturs.
Circumstantiality	Responding to a question in an indirect and delayed manner. The patient brings in many unnecessary and tedious details.
Pressured speech	Increasingly spontaneous speech in which the patient speaks loudly and rapidly and is difficult to interrupt. This pattern of speech often is seen in mania.
Distractible speech	Abrupt cessation of speech in the middle of a sentence or idea and change in subject, often in response to a nearby stimulus.
Clanging	A pattern of speech in which sounds govern word choice, often through use of redundant or rhyming word choices.

Catatonic Motor Behaviors

Catatonic symptoms should only be considered present when they are obvious and have been directly observed by the clinician or other professional (Table 2–4).

Inappropriate Affect

The patient's affect expressed is inappropriate or incongruous, not simply flat or blunted. This may take the form of smiling or assuming a silly facial expression while talking about a serious or sad subject.

TABLE 2–4. Features of catatonic motor behaviors

Stupor	The patient has a marked decrease in reactivity to the environment and reduction of spontaneous movements and activity. The patient might appear to be unaware of the nature of his or her surroundings.
Rigidity	The patient shows signs of motor rigidity (e.g., resistance to passive movement).
Waxy flexibility (catalepsy)	The patient maintains postures that he or she is placed for at least 15 seconds.
Excitement	The patient has apparently purposeless and stereotyped excited motor activity not influenced by external stimuli.
Posturing and mannerisms	The patient voluntarily assumes an inappropriate or a bizarre posture. These involve movements or gestures that appear artificial or contrived, are not appropriate to the situation, or are stereotyped and repetitive.

Alogia (Poverty of Speech, Poverty of Content of Speech)

Alogia refers to impoverished thinking and cognition that often occurs in patients with schizophrenia. Patients with alogia display thinking processes that seem empty, turgid, or slow. Table 2–5 describes the various types of alogia.

Affective Flattening or Blunting

Affective flattening (or blunting) manifests as a characteristic impoverishment of emotional expression, reactivity, and feeling.

Unchanging facial expression. The patient's face does not change expression, or changes less than is normally expected, as the emotional content of the discourse changes.

Decreased spontaneous movements. The patient sits quietly throughout the interview and shows few or no spontaneous movements.

Paucity of expressive gestures. The patient does not use his or her body as an aid for expressing ideas through means such as hand gestures, sitting forward in the chair when intent on a subject, or leaning back when relaxed.

TABLE 2–5. Types of alogia

Poverty of speech	The patient has a restricted amount of spontaneous speech, so that replies to questions tend to be brief, concrete, and unelaborated.
Poverty of content of speech	Although the patient's replies are long enough so that the amount of speech is adequate, the speech conveys little information. Language tends to be vague, repetitive, and stereotyped.
Blocking	The patient's train of speech is interrupted before a thought or an idea has been completed. After a period of silence, which may last from a few seconds to minutes, the person indicates that he or she cannot recall what he or she has been saying or meant to say.
Increased latency of response	The patient takes a longer time to reply to questions than is considered normal.
Perseveration	The patient persistently repeats words, ideas, or phrases so that once the patient begins to use a particular word, he or she continually returns to it while speaking.

Poor eye contact. The patient avoids looking at others or using his or her eyes as an aid for expression. He or she appears to be staring into space even while talking.

Lack of vocal inflections. The patient fails to show normal vocal emphasis patterns. Speech has a monotonic quality, and important words are not emphasized through changes in pitch or volume.

Avolition–Apathy

Avolition–apathy manifests as a characteristic lack of energy and drive. Patients become inert and are unable to mobilize themselves to initiate or persist in completing many different kinds of tasks.

Grooming and hygiene. The patient pays less attention to grooming and hygiene than is normal. Clothing may appear sloppy, outdated, or soiled. He or she may bathe infrequently, and this may lead to greasy or uncombed hair, dirty hands, body odor, or unclean teeth and bad breath.

Impersistence at work or school. The patient has difficulty seeking or maintaining employment (or doing schoolwork) as appropriate for his or her age and gender.

- Have you been able to (work, go to school) during the past month?
- Have you been attending vocational rehabilitation or occupational therapy sessions (in the hospital)?

Physical anergia. The patient tends to be physically inert; he or she may sit in a chair for hours at a time. If encouraged to become involved in an activity, the patient might participate only briefly and then wander away or disengage and return to sitting alone.

- How have you been spending your time?
- Do you have any trouble getting yourself going?

Anhedonia–Asociality

Anhedonia–asociality might manifest as a loss of interest in pleasurable activities, an inability to experience pleasure when participating in activities normally considered pleasurable, or a lack of involvement in social relationships of various kinds.

Recreational interests and activities. The patient might have few or no interests, activities, or hobbies. Although this symptom could begin insidiously or slowly, there usually will be some obvious decline from an earlier level of interest and activity.

- What do you do for enjoyment?
- Have you been attending recreational therapy?

Sexual interest and activity. The patient might show decreased sexual interest and sexual activity or enjoyment compared with what would be judged healthy for the patient's age and marital status.

- What has your sex drive been like?
- Have you been able to enjoy sex lately?
- When was the last time you engaged in sexual activity?

Ability to feel intimacy and closeness. The patient might not be able to form intimate and close relationships appropriate for his or her age, gender, and family status.

- Do you feel close to your family (husband, wife, partner, children)?
- Is there anyone outside your family to whom you feel especially close?

Relationships with friends and peers.   Patients also might be relatively restricted in their relationships with friends and peers of either gender.

- Do you have many friends?
- Have you gotten to know any patients in the hospital?

Attention

The patient may have trouble focusing attention or could only focus sporadically and erratically.

Social inattentiveness.   While involved in social situations or activities, the patient appears inattentive. He or she looks away during conversations, does not pick up the topic during a discussion, or appears uninvolved or disengaged.

Manic Symptoms

Euphoric Mood

The patient has had one or more distinct periods of euphoric, irritable, or expansive mood not caused by alcohol or drug intoxication.

- Have you been feeling too good or even high—clearly different from your normal self?
- Have you felt irritable and easily annoyed?

Increase in Activity

The patient shows an increase in involvement or activity level associated with work, family, friends, sex drive, new projects, interests, or activities (e.g., telephone calls, letter writing).

- Are you more active or involved in things compared with the way you usually are?
- Have you been unable to sit still, or have you had to be moving or pacing back and forth?

Racing Thoughts/Flight of Ideas

The patient has the subjective experience that his or her thinking is markedly accelerated. For example, "My thoughts are ahead of my speech."

- Have your thoughts been racing through your mind?
- Do you have more ideas than usual?

Inflated Self-Esteem

The patient has increased self-esteem and appraisal of his or her worth, contacts, influence, power, or knowledge (might be delusional) compared with his or her usual level.

- Do you feel more self-confident than usual?
- Do you feel that you are especially important or that you have special talents or abilities?

Decreased Need for Sleep

The patient needs less sleep than usual to feel rested.

- Do you need less sleep than usual to feel rested?

Distractibility

The patient's attention is too easily drawn to unimportant or irrelevant external stimuli.

- Are you easily distracted by things around you?

Poor Judgment

The patient shows excessive involvement in activities that have a high potential for painful consequences (e.g., buying sprees, sexual indiscretions, foolish business investments).

- Have you done anything that caused trouble for you or your family or friends?
- Have you done anything foolish with money?
- Have you done anything sexually that was unusual for you?

Depressive Symptoms

Dysphoric Mood

The patient feels sad, despondent, discouraged, or unhappy; significant anxiety or tense irritability also should be rated as a dysphoric mood.

- Have you been having periods of feeling depressed, sad, or hopeless? When you didn't care about anything or couldn't enjoy anything?
- Have you felt tense, anxious, or irritable?

Change in Appetite or Weight

The patient has had significant weight change. The weight change should not include change due to intentional dieting.

- Have you had any changes in your appetite—either increased or decreased?
- Have you lost or gained much more weight than is usual for you?

Insomnia or Hypersomnia

Patterns of insomnia include *initial* (trouble going to sleep), *middle* (waking in the middle of the night but eventually falling asleep), and *terminal* (waking early—e.g., 2:00 A.M. to 5:00 A.M.—and remaining awake).

- Have you had trouble sleeping?
- Have you been sleeping more than usual?
- How much sleep do you typically get in a 24-hour period?

Psychomotor Agitation

The patient is unable to sit still, with a need to keep moving. Objective evidence (e.g., hand wringing, fidgeting, pacing) should be present.

- Have you felt restless or agitated?
- Do you have trouble sitting still?

Psychomotor Retardation

The patient feels slowed down and experiences great difficulty moving. (Objective evidence [e.g., slowed speech] should be present.)

- Have you been feeling slowed down?

Loss of Interest or Pleasure

The patient has loss of interest or pleasure in usual activities or a decrease in sexual drive.

- Have you noticed a change in your interest in things you normally enjoy?

Loss of Energy

The patient has a loss of energy, becomes easily fatigued, or feels tired.

- Have you had a tendency to feel more tired than usual?

Feelings of Worthlessness

In addition to feelings of worthlessness, the patient might report feelings of self-reproach or excessive or inappropriate guilt.

- Have you been feeling down on yourself?
- Have you been feeling guilty about anything?

Diminished Ability to Think or Concentrate

The patient complains of diminished ability to think or concentrate, such as slowed thinking or indecisiveness, not associated with marked derailment or incoherence.

- Have you had trouble thinking?
- Have you had trouble making decisions?

Recurrent Thoughts of Death/Suicide

The patient has thoughts about death and dying, plus possible wishes to be dead or to take his or her life.

- Have you been thinking about death or taking your own life?

Distinct Quality to Mood

The patient's depressed mood is experienced as distinctly different from the type of feelings experienced after the death of a loved one.

- The feelings of (sadness) you are having now, are they the same as the feelings you would have had when someone close to you died, or are they different?

Nonreactivity of Mood

The patient does not feel much better, even temporarily, when something good happens.

- Do your feelings of depression go away or get better when you do something you enjoy?

Diurnal Variation

The patient's mood shifts during the course of the day. Some patients feel bad in the morning, then gradually improve, and others describe the reverse.

- Is there any time of the day that is especially bad for you?

Anxiety Symptoms

Panic Attacks

The patient has discrete episodes of intense fear or discomfort in which a variety of symptoms occur, such as shortness of breath, dizziness, palpitations, or shaking.

- Have you ever experienced a sudden attack of panic or fear in which you felt extremely uncomfortable?

Agoraphobia

The patient has a fear of places or situations from which escape might be difficult.

- Have you ever been afraid of going outside, so that you tended to just stay home all the time?
- Have you been afraid of getting caught or trapped somewhere so that you would be unable to escape?

Social Anxiety

The patient has a fear of being in a social situation in which he or she will be seen by others and could do something that he or she might find humiliating or embarrassing.

- Do you have any special fears, such as a fear of public speaking, or eating in front of others?

Specific Phobia

The patient is afraid of some specific stimulus, such as animals (e.g., snakes, insects), blood, high places, or flying.

- Are you afraid of snakes? Blood? Air travel?

Obsessions

The patient experiences persistent ideas, thoughts, or impulses that are unwanted and experienced as unpleasant. The patient tends to ruminate and worry about them.

- Are you ever bothered by persistent ideas that you can't get out of your head, such as being dirty or contaminated?

Compulsions

The patient has to perform specific acts over and over in a way that he or she recognizes as senseless or inappropriate.

The compulsions are usually performed to ease some worry or to prevent a feared event.

- Are there any types of actions that you have to perform over and over, such as washing your hands or checking the stove?

Further Reading

American Psychiatric Association: Pocket Guide to Psychiatric Evaluation of Adults. Arlington, VA, American Psychiatric Association Publishing, 2017

Andreasen NC: Thought, language, and communication disorders, I: clinical assessment, definition of terms, and evaluation of their reliability. Arch Gen Psychiatry 36(12):1315–1321, 1979

Chisholm MS, Lyketsos CG: Systematic Psychiatric Evaluation: A Step-by-Step Guide to Applying the Perspectives of Psychiatry. Baltimore, MD, Johns Hopkins University Press, 2012

Folstein MF, Folstein SE, McHugh PR: "Mini-mental state": a practical method for grading the cognitive state of patients for the clinician. J Psychiatr Res 12(3):189–198, 1975

MacKinnon RA, Michels R, Buckley PJ: The Psychiatric Interview in Clinical Practice, 3rd Edition. Arlington, VA, American Psychiatric Association Publishing, 2016

Nasreddine ZS, Phillips NA, Bédirian V, et al: The Montreal Cognitive Assessment, MoCA: a brief screening tool for mild cognitive impairment. J Am Geriatr Soc 53(4):695–699, 2005

Shea SC: Psychiatric Interviewing: The Art of Understanding. A Practical Guide for Psychiatrists, Psychologists, Counselors, Social Workers, Nurses, and Other Mental Health Professionals, 3rd Edition. Philadelphia, PA, WB Saunders, 2016

PART II

Psychiatric Disorders

Chapter 3

Neurodevelopmental (Child) Disorders

DSM-5 has specified a group of disorders that typically *arise* rather than simply *occur* during childhood and adolescence. Among many changes, the umbrella diagnosis *autism spectrum disorder* (ASD) was created by merging autistic disorder, Rett's disorder, childhood disintegrative disorder, and Asperger's disorder. The change was prompted by research showing that these disorders were not independent and that clinicians had difficulty distinguishing them. The DSM-5 neurodevelopmental disorders are listed in Table 3–1.

Child psychiatry is one of the most challenging and interesting areas of specialization within psychiatry. Approximately 5%–15% of children will experience a psychiatric disturbance severe enough to require treatment or impair their functioning during the course of a year. Because the child psychiatrist must know a great deal about other childhood illnesses, maturation processes, and developmental disorders, the field is closely allied with pediatrics and requires a good knowledge of general medicine. Furthermore, a clinician working in child psychiatry has an opportunity to catch disorders at their earliest stage.

In this chapter, we review disorders most frequently seen in child psychiatry clinics or in a family practice setting. These include the following:

- Intellectual disability
- Communication disorders
- Autism spectrum disorder
- Attention-deficit/hyperactivity disorder (ADHD)
- Specific learning disorder
- Motor disorders (including tic disorders)

TABLE 3–1. DSM-5 neurodevelopmental disorders

Intellectual disabilities

Intellectual disability (intellectual developmental disorder)

Global developmental delay

Communication disorders

Language disorder

Speech sound disorder

Childhood-onset fluency disorder (stuttering)

Social (pragmatic) communication disorder

Autism spectrum disorder

Attention-deficit/hyperactivity disorder

Specific learning disorder

Motor disorders

Developmental coordination disorder

Stereotypic movement disorder

Tic disorders

    Tourette's disorder

    Persistent (chronic) motor or vocal tic disorder

    Provisional tic disorder

Assessment of Children

Assessment of children requires an understanding of special techniques and the importance of flexible norms or criteria, involvement of family or significant others, and increased role of nonphysicians in the health care team.

With children, it is important to emphasize a developmental approach that accounts for the growth and maturation processes that children undergo and assesses each individual child in light of his or her specific life situation and strengths and weaknesses. As you evaluate the child, ask yourself the following questions:

• What level of emotional and intellectual maturity does this child have?

- What are his or her particular strengths?
- How do they provide a protective and healing element?
- What specific weaknesses are present?
- What stresses are affecting the child?
- How do those stresses affect him or her at this particular stage of life?
- How do gender-specific challenges affect expression of illness and its treatment?

Who Is the Patient?

Children typically are referred by parents, other caregivers, or the courts. The child might be unwilling, noncompliant, distrusting, or resentful, which makes assessment challenging. Although the child usually will be the identified patient, it could become clear that the parents themselves have serious problems. It may be necessary to reassess the situation and to suggest treatment for the parents in addition to—or even instead of—the child.

Assessment of the Child

Childhood disorders can be diagnosed in individuals ranging from infants through those in their late teens or early 20s. Obviously, the standard approaches to interviewing and assessment described in Chapter 2 do not apply well to infants, children, or young teenagers. For example, young children might not be able to respond to questions about concepts such as depression, loneliness, or anger. The interviewer needs to talk to children at a much more concrete level, asking questions such as

- Do you feel like crying? Why?
- Do you ever want to hit people? Whom?
- Who are your best friends?
- How often do you see them?
- What kinds of things do you do together?

In addition to interviewing the child and parents or caregivers, playing games with the child often provides some insight into the child's ability to function interpersonally, to tolerate frustration, or to focus his or her attention. Imaginative play or use of dolls that can represent important figures in the child's life also might give the clinician some sense as to the patient's feelings toward others and relationships. Taking turns telling stories can be a way to elicit information as well. Direct observation of activity level, motor skills, verbal expression, and vocabulary also is a fundamental component of assessment. Observing the child's behavior could help compensate for the limited reliability of symptom reporting in very young children.

Involvement of Family and Others

Clinicians who work with children usually need to work with their families and significant others as well. The degree of family involvement varies, of course, depending on the age of the child. With very young children, the parents likely are the primary informants and important recipients of treatment as well. For grade-school children, involvement of family members is essential, but the child becomes an increasingly valuable participant in both assessment and treatment. Teenagers usually are at the forefront of the assessment and treatment process, although the family will provide resources much of the time. Whether to maintain complete confidentiality or to share information becomes a critical issue when assessing teenagers. In general, the clinician should assure teenagers that what they tell the clinician will remain there, unless the teenager gives permission to share the information. Only in situations dangerous to the child, such as a clear risk of suicide, should a clinician breach confidentiality.

Child psychiatry often involves the participation of a health care team that could include, in addition to the psychiatrist, a social worker, an educational specialist, and a psychologist who develops programs for behavioral management, might do psychotherapy, and may work with the child, family, and school system.

Psychological and Educational Testing

Psychological and educational testing often plays a central role in the evaluation of children. Tests that are commonly used in child psychiatry are listed in Table 3–2.

Physical Examination

In addition to the standard physical examination, the clinician should inspect the child for indications of congenital

TABLE 3–2. Cognitive, psychological, and educational tests commonly used in child psychiatry

Factor	Test
Intelligence	Stanford-Binet Intelligence Scale
	Wechsler Intelligence Scale for Children (WISC-IV)
	Peabody Picture Vocabulary Test
	Kaufman ABC
	Wechsler Preschool and Primary Scale of Intelligence (WPPSI)
Educational achievement	Iowa Test of Basic Skills (ITBS)
	Iowa Test of Educational Development (ITED)
	Wide Range Achievement Test—Revised (WRAT-R)
Adaptive behavior	Vineland Adaptive Behavior Scales
	Conners' Teacher Rating Scale—Revised
Perceptual-motor abilities	Draw-a-Person Test
	Bender-Gestalt
	Benton Visual Retention Test
	Purdue Pegboard Test
	Beery Developmental Test of Visual-Motor Integration

anomalies, such as a high-arched palate, low-set ears, single palmar creases, unusual carrying angle, webbing, abnormalities of the genitalia, and neuroectodermal anomalies. Such anomalies could suggest obtaining a magnetic resonance imaging scan to assess for the presence of structural brain abnormalities, particularly in the midline. The clinician should also be attentive to assessment of neurological soft signs in children, such as graphesthesia, left–right discrimination, motor coordination, and simple perceptual-motor skills.

Intellectual Disability (Intellectual Developmental Disorder)

Intellectual disability (intellectual developmental disorder [IDD]), formerly *mental retardation*, is characterized by deficits in general mental abilities and impairment in everyday adaptive functioning with onset in the early developmental period. The diagnosis no longer relies on the presence of an IQ less than 70. Rather, emphasis is on adaptive functioning—that is, how well the person functions in terms of social and behavioral interactions, conceptual and intellectual life, and practical day-to-day living skills. Nevertheless, measuring intelligence remains a critical part of the assessment of the person's intellectual functioning. IDD is rated as mild, moderate, severe, or profound. The DSM-5 criteria for intellectual developmental disorder are provided Box 3–1.

Box 3–1.   DSM-5 Criteria for Intellectual Disability (Intellectual Developmental Disorder)

Intellectual disability (intellectual developmental disorder) is a disorder with onset during the developmental period that includes both intellectual and adaptive functioning deficits in conceptual, social, and practical domains. The following three criteria must be met:

A. Deficits in intellectual functions, such as reasoning, problem solving, planning, abstract thinking, judgment, academic learning, and learning from experience, confirmed by both clinical assessment and individualized, standardized intelligence testing.
B. Deficits in adaptive functioning that result in failure to meet developmental and sociocultural standards for personal independence and social responsibility. Without ongoing support, the adaptive deficits limit functioning in one or more activities of daily life, such as communication, social participation, and independent living, across multiple environments, such as home, school, work, and community.
C. Onset of intellectual and adaptive deficits during the developmental period.

Note: The diagnostic term *intellectual disability* is the equivalent term for the ICD-11 diagnosis of *intellectual developmental disorders*. Although the term *intellectual disability* is used throughout this manual, both terms are used in the title to clarify relationships with other classification systems. Moreover, a federal statute in the United States (Public Law 111-256, Rosa's Law) replaces the term *mental retardation* with *intellectual disability,* and research journals use the term *intellectual disability.* Thus, *intellectual disability* is the term in common use by medical, educational, and other professions and by the lay public and advocacy groups.

Specify current severity:
Mild
Moderate
Severe
Profound

Standardized intelligence testing usually involves IQ measurement. With such tests, the category of intellectual disability is considered to be approximately two standard deviations or more below the population mean, including a margin for error (approximately ±5 points).

Deficits in *adaptive functioning* also are assessed to determine how well a person meets community standards of personal independence and social responsibility in three critical domains:

- *Conceptual (academic):* competence in memory, language, reading, writing, math reasoning, and acquisition of practical knowledge; problem solving; and judgment in novel situations; among others.
- *Social:* awareness of others' thoughts, feelings, and experiences; empathy; interpersonal communication skills; friendship abilities; and social judgment; among others.
- *Practical:* learning and self-management across life settings, including personal care, job responsibilities, money management, recreation, self-management of behavior, and school and work task organization, among others.

Children with *mild* IDD represent most cases, constituting approximately 85% of identified individuals. These children are considered educable and are usually able to attend special classes and work toward the long-term goal of being able to function in the community and to hold a job. Children with *moderate* IDD constitute approximately 10% of the intellectually disabled population. They are considered trainable, in that they can learn to talk, recognize their name and other simple words, perform activities of self-care such as bathing or doing their laundry, and handle small change. They require management and treatment in special education classes. Children with *severe* and *profound* IDD constitute the smallest groups. Individuals in these categories usually need institutional care.

Epidemiology and Clinical Findings

IDD affects approximately 1%–2% of the general population. It is more common in males, with a male-to-female ratio of approximately 2:1. Mild disorder is more common in the lower socioeconomic classes, but cases of moderate, severe, and profound intellectual disability are equally common among all social classes.

Long-term outcome is variable. Some severe and profound forms may be associated with progressive physical deterioration and premature death, as early as the teens or early 20s (e.g., Tay-Sachs disease). Individuals with mild and moderate disorders have a somewhat reduced life expectancy, but active intervention could enhance their quality of life. Similar to all children, children with IDD might show maturational spurts that could not have been predicted at an earlier age. Typically, these children progress through normal milestones, such as sitting, standing, talking, and learning numbers and letters, in a pattern similar to that of nondisabled children but at a slower rate.

Etiology and Pathophysiology

IDD represents a final common pathway produced by a variety of factors that injure the brain and affect its normal development. Individuals with moderate to profound impairment often have an identifiable cause for their IDD, whereas those with mild impairment might not and probably the disorder develops through complex multifactorial combinations. *Down syndrome* (trisomy 21) is the most common chromosomal cause of IDD. *Fragile X syndrome* is the most common heritable form of IDD and is second only to Down syndrome in frequency. The fragile X gene contains an unstable segment that expands as it is passed through generations and affects children differently depending on whether it is passed through fathers or mothers (imprinting). Inborn errors of metabolism account for a small percentage of cases; examples include Tay-Sachs disease and untreated phenylketonuria.

In addition to these clearly defined genetic causes, a substantial portion of cases of IDD might also reflect polygenic inheritance, possibly interacting with nongenetic factors such as nutrition and psychosocial nurturance. Many prenatal factors also could affect fetal development and lead to neurodevelopmental anomalies. The high rate of Down syndrome in children born to older mothers is a prime example. Other prenatal factors that could affect fetal development include maternal malnutrition or substance abuse; exposure to mutagens such as radiation; maternal illnesses such as diabetes, toxemia, or rubella; and maternal abuse and neglect. *Fetal alcohol syndrome* is a common nongenetic cause of IDD. Perinatal and early postnatal factors also may contribute and include the following:

- Traumatic deliveries that cause brain injury
- Malnutrition
- Exposure to toxins
- Infections such as encephalitis
- Head injuries occurring during infancy or early childhood

Differential Diagnosis

The differential diagnosis of IDD (particularly mild impairment) can be complex because of frequent comorbidity of other childhood disorders including ADHD, learning disorders, autism spectrum disorder, and childhood psychoses or mood disorders. Seizure disorders also are common in these children.

Clinical Management

A comprehensive treatment plan should be developed to determine the best situation in which to place and treat the child—one that takes into account the needs and abilities of both the child and the parents. Decisions range from care in the home (supplemented by family support and special education), to placement in a foster or group home, to long-term institutionalization. Because most children with IDD are mildly affected, most will remain at home, at least initially. Because the parents of some of these children themselves have IDD, ongoing evaluation through social service agencies might be helpful and even necessary to ensure the child's needs are being met.

Communication Disorders

Communication disorders interfere with a child's ability to communicate their needs, desires, and emotions. Although not traditionally considered psychiatric disorders, they cause distress and impair the child's ability to function and are important for purposes of differential diagnosis. The communication disorders are as follows:

Language disorder: a persistent disturbance in the development and use of spoken language, written language, or sign language because of deficits in comprehension or production.

Speech sound disorder: persistent difficulties in speech production that are developmentally inappropriate, such as articulation, fluency, and voice production.

Childhood-onset fluency disorder (stuttering): a disturbance in the normal fluency and time patterning of speech that is inappropriate for the child's age.

Social (pragmatic) communication disorder: difficulty with the social use of verbal and nonverbal communication.

Autism Spectrum Disorder

ASD is a disorder whose essential features are persistent impairment in reciprocal social communication and social interaction, combined with restricted, repetitive patterns of behavior, interests, or activities. Present from infancy or early childhood, the disorder might not be detected until later because of minimal social demands and support from parents or caregivers in early years. When using DSM-5 criteria, the clinician can specify the child's condition by indicating his or her overall symptom severity and intellectual and/or language impairment, and noting whether there is a known genetic disorder, epilepsy, or comorbid intellectual disability. For example, rather than receiving a diagnosis of DSM-IV Asperger's disorder, the child now has "autism spectrum disorder, without accompanying intellectual impairment and without accompanying language impairment." The DSM-5 criteria for ASD are presented in Box 3–2.

Box 3–2.   DSM-5 Criteria for Autism Spectrum Disorder

A. Persistent deficits in social communication and social interaction across multiple contexts, as manifested by all of the following, currently or by history (examples are illustrative, not exhaustive; see text):

1. Deficits in social-emotional reciprocity, ranging, for example, from abnormal social approach and failure of normal

back-and-forth conversation; to reduced sharing of interests, emotions, or affect; to failure to initiate or respond to social interactions.

2. Deficits in nonverbal communicative behaviors used for social interaction, ranging, for example, from poorly integrated verbal and nonverbal communication; to abnormalities in eye contact and body language or deficits in understanding and use of gestures; to a total lack of facial expressions and nonverbal communication.

3. Deficits in developing, maintaining, and understanding relationships, ranging, for example, from difficulties adjusting behavior to suit various social contexts; to difficulties in sharing imaginative play or in making friends; to absence of interest in peers.

Specify current severity:

Severity is based on social communication impairments and restricted, repetitive patterns of behavior.

B. Restricted, repetitive patterns of behavior, interests, or activities, as manifested by at least two of the following, currently or by history (examples are illustrative, not exhaustive; see text):

1. Stereotyped or repetitive motor movements, use of objects, or speech (e.g., simple motor stereotypies, lining up toys or flipping objects, echolalia, idiosyncratic phrases).

2. Insistence on sameness, inflexible adherence to routines, or ritualized patterns of verbal or nonverbal behavior (e.g., extreme distress at small changes, difficulties with transitions, rigid thinking patterns, greeting rituals, need to take same route or eat same food every day).

3. Highly restricted, fixated interests that are abnormal in intensity or focus (e.g., strong attachment to or preoccupation with unusual objects, excessively circumscribed or perseverative interests).

4. Hyper- or hyporeactivity to sensory input or unusual interest in sensory aspects of the environment (e.g., apparent indifference to pain/temperature, adverse response to specific sounds or textures, excessive smelling or touching of objects, visual fascination with lights or movement).

Specify current severity:

Severity is based on social communication impairments and restricted, repetitive patterns of behavior.

C. Symptoms must be present in the early developmental period (but may not become fully manifest until social demands exceed limited capacities, or may be masked by learned strategies in later life).

D. Symptoms cause clinically significant impairment in social, occupational, or other important areas of current functioning.

E. These disturbances are not better explained by intellectual disability (intellectual developmental disorder) or global developmental delay. Intellectual disability and autism spectrum disorder frequently co-occur; to make comorbid diagnoses of autism spectrum disorder and intellectual disability, social communication should be below that expected for general developmental level.

Note: Individuals with a well-established DSM-IV diagnosis of autistic disorder, Asperger's disorder, or pervasive developmental disorder not otherwise specified should be given the diagnosis of autism spectrum disorder. Individuals who have marked deficits in social communication, but whose symptoms do not otherwise meet criteria for autism spectrum disorder, should be evaluated for social (pragmatic) communication disorder.

Clinical Findings

Symptoms vary greatly depending on syndrome severity, the child's age, and his or her developmental level. For those with a more severe disorder, within the child's first 3–6 months of life, the parents might note that the child has not developed a normal pattern of smiling or responding to cuddling. The first clear sign of abnormality usually is in language. As the child grows older, he or she does not progress through developmental milestones such as learning to say words and speak sentences. The failure to develop spoken language typically is what leads parents to seek medical attention. Verbal impairments range from the complete absence of verbal speech to mildly deviant speech and language patterns. Severely affected children also might appear to lack the ability to bond with their parents or with others. In milder cases, they have some interaction but lack warmth, sensitivity, and awareness.

Finally, the child's behavioral repertoire is impaired. There is an intense and rigid commitment to maintaining specific routines, and severely affected children tend to become quite distressed if routines are interrupted. They might have to sit in a specific chair, dress in a particular way, or eat specific foods.

Most persons with severe ASD show some evidence of IDD, but others have normal intelligence. Some have very specific talents or abilities, particularly in music or mathematics.

Epidemiology and Course

ASD affects approximately 1% of the general population, but severe cases are less common. More boys than girls are affected, with a ratio of about 4:1. Onset is early, with problems typically noted during the first or second year of life. For most children with severe ASD, the disorder is chronic and lifelong. Some will show improvement as they mature, whereas others might worsen. Few are able to progress normally through school or live independently. Nearly all of the defining features of the disorder, including social aloofness, language abnormalities, and rigid and ritualistic behavior, tend to persist into adulthood. Good prognostic features include higher IQ and better language and social skills.

Etiology and Pathophysiology

ASD is highly heritable, as shown in family and twin studies. IDD and both speech and language disorders run in these families as well. Approximately 15% of cases are associated with a known genetic mechanism.

Imaging studies show that children with ASD have large brain size relative to body size, with some evidence for gyral malformation. Abnormalities in the cerebellum (particularly the vermis), the temporal lobes, and the hippocampal complex, as well as cerebral asymmetries, also have been reported. Functional imaging studies suggest the presence of an overall impairment in connectivity in brain networks used for attention, consciousness, and self-awareness. Neuropathological studies have reported small, densely packed—and presumably immature—cells in limbic structures in the cerebellum. Physically, these children have a variety of soft neurological signs and primitive reflexes, an excess of non-right-handedness, and an apparent failure to achieve normal cerebral dominance of language functions in the left hemisphere.

Differential Diagnosis

Children with symptoms suggestive of ASD should be screened for other disorders such as phenylketonuria or Down syndrome. Because these children present with profound social withdrawal, check hearing and vision to rule out sensory defects as a cause. Order electroencephalography when comorbid seizure disorders are suspected. IQ testing will help assess the child's intellectual strengths and weaknesses.

The major differential diagnoses include childhood psychosis, IDD, communication disorders, and selective mutism. The distinction between ASD and schizophrenia rests on the presence of overt psychotic symptoms such as delusions and hallucinations. The distinction with IDD can be difficult. Children with IDD typically have pervasive intellectual impairments, whereas children with ASD tend to have a much more uneven profile of functional intellectual abilities and might be normal to superior in some areas. Rule out selective mutism; in these cases, the child fails to speak despite an ability to do so, and he or she has none of the cardinal features of ASD.

Clinical Management

Children who are severely affected need special education or specialized day care programs that emphasize improvement in social and language skills. Medications often are used as adjuncts to these supportive and behavioral approaches. Children with seizures require anticonvulsants. Antipsychotics have been found to decrease aggressive and stereotypical patterns of behavior. The second-generation antipsychotics risperidone and aripiprazole are U.S. Food and Drug Administration (FDA)–approved for treating irritability in ASD. Other medications that might be helpful are selective serotonin reuptake inhibitors for individuals with depression, anxiety, or obsessive-compulsive symptoms, and stimulants for those with symptoms of inattention or hyperactivity.

Attention-Deficit/Hyperactivity Disorder

ADHD is one of the most common disorders that child psychiatrists diagnose and treat. Children with ADHD are physically overactive, distractible, inattentive, impulsive, and difficult to manage. ADHD typically is evident early in childhood, with signs of increased activity being noted very early. The disorder can persist into adulthood. ADHD is defined by two broad groups of symptoms: 1) inattention and 2) hyperactivity/impulsivity. Subtypes can be specified to indicate whether the presentation is predominantly inattentive, predominantly hyperactive/impulsive, or mixed. The DSM-5 criteria for ADHD are shown in Box 3–3.

Box 3–3. DSM-5 Criteria for Attention-Deficit/ Hyperactivity Disorder

A. A persistent pattern of inattention and/or hyperactivity-impulsivity that interferes with functioning or development, as characterized by (1) and/or (2):

1. **Inattention:** Six (or more) of the following symptoms have persisted for at least 6 months to a degree that is inconsistent with developmental level and that negatively impacts directly on social and academic/occupational activities:

   Note: The symptoms are not solely a manifestation of oppositional behavior, defiance, hostility, or failure to understand tasks or instructions. For older adolescents and adults (age 17 and older), at least five symptoms are required.

   a. Often fails to give close attention to details or makes careless mistakes in schoolwork, at work, or during other activities (e.g., overlooks or misses details, work is inaccurate).

   b. Often has difficulty sustaining attention in tasks or play activities (e.g., has difficulty remaining focused during lectures, conversations, or lengthy reading).

   c. Often does not seem to listen when spoken to directly (e.g., mind seems elsewhere, even in the absence of any obvious distraction).

   d. Often does not follow through on instructions and fails to finish schoolwork, chores, or duties in the workplace (e.g., starts tasks but quickly loses focus and is easily sidetracked).

   e. Often has difficulty organizing tasks and activities (e.g., difficulty managing sequential tasks; difficulty keeping materials and belongings in order; messy, disorganized work; has poor time management; fails to meet deadlines).

   f. Often avoids, dislikes, or is reluctant to engage in tasks that require sustained mental effort (e.g., schoolwork or homework; for older adolescents and adults, preparing reports, completing forms, reviewing lengthy papers).

   g. Often loses things necessary for tasks or activities (e.g., school materials, pencils, books, tools, wallets, keys, paperwork, eyeglasses, mobile telephones).

   h. Is often easily distracted by extraneous stimuli (for older adolescents and adults, may include unrelated thoughts).

Neurodevelopmental (Child) Disorders

    i.   Is often forgetful in daily activities (e.g., doing chores, running errands; for older adolescents and adults, returning calls, paying bills, keeping appointments).

2. **Hyperactivity and impulsivity:** Six (or more) of the following symptoms have persisted for at least 6 months to a degree that is inconsistent with developmental level and that negatively impacts directly on social and academic/occupational activities:

   Note: The symptoms are not solely a manifestation of oppositional behavior, defiance, hostility, or a failure to understand tasks or instructions. For older adolescents and adults (age 17 and older), at least five symptoms are required.

   a.   Often fidgets with or taps hands or feet or squirms in seat.

   b.   Often leaves seat in situations when remaining seated is expected (e.g., leaves his or her place in the classroom, in the office or other workplace, or in other situations that require remaining in place).

   c.   Often runs about or climbs in situations where it is inappropriate. (**Note:** In adolescents or adults, may be limited to feeling restless.)

   d.   Often unable to play or engage in leisure activities quietly.

   e.   Is often "on the go," acting as if "driven by a motor" (e.g., is unable to be or uncomfortable being still for extended time, as in restaurants, meetings; may be experienced by others as being restless or difficult to keep up with).

   f.   Often talks excessively.

   g.   Often blurts out an answer before a question has been completed (e.g., completes people's sentences; cannot wait for turn in conversation).

   h.   Often has difficulty waiting his or her turn (e.g., while waiting in line).

   i.   Often interrupts or intrudes on others (e.g., butts into conversations, games, or activities; may start using other people's things without asking or receiving permission; for adolescents and adults, may intrude into or take over what others are doing).

B. Several inattentive or hyperactive-impulsive symptoms were present prior to age 12 years.

C. Several inattentive or hyperactive-impulsive symptoms are present in two or more settings (e.g., at home, school, or work; with friends or relatives; in other activities).

D. There is clear evidence that the symptoms interfere with, or reduce the quality of, social, academic, or occupational functioning.

E. The symptoms do not occur exclusively during the course of schizophrenia or another psychotic disorder and are not better explained by another mental disorder (e.g., mood disorder, anxiety disorder, dissociative disorder, personality disorder, substance intoxication or withdrawal).

Epidemiology and Clinical Findings

The prevalence of ADHD is about 5% in children and 2.5% in adults. It is more common in boys than in girls, with a male-to-female ratio of approximately 3:1. Approximately one-half of the children with this disorder have a good outcome, completing school on schedule with acceptable grades consistent with their family background and family expectations. Longitudinal studies show that a substantial portion of children with ADHD remain relatively impaired into adulthood. With adults, inattentiveness persists as hyperactivity subsides.

Etiology and Pathophysiology

ADHD runs in families and appears to be highly heritable. Genetic studies have begun to identify genes underlying ADHD, but none appear causal. Nongenetic factors also may be important in the development of ADHD. Risk factors include perinatal problems such as maternal smoking, substance abuse, obstetrical complications, malnutrition, exposure to toxins, and viral infections.

Brain imaging studies indicate that the prefrontal cortex, basal ganglia, and cerebellum either are reduced in size or have abnormalities in asymmetry. Neuropsychological data show that individuals with ADHD have difficulties with response inhibition, executive functions mediated through the prefrontal cortex, or timing functions mediated through the cerebellum. Functional imaging studies have shown hypoperfusion in prefrontal and basal ganglia regions that might be reversible with stimulant treatment.

Differential Diagnosis

Comorbid disorders are common among children with ADHD, including seizure disorders, conduct disorder, oppositional defiant disorder, and learning disorders. Childhood bipolar disorder or depression could manifest with similar or overlapping symptoms. ADHD symptoms might appear to be a normal response to an abusive home environment.

Clinical Management

Stimulants such as methylphenidate and amphetamine salts are considered first-line treatments for ADHD. Other options include atomoxetine (Strattera), guanfacine (Intuniv), and clonidine (Kapvay). In general, methylphenidate and dextroamphetamine offer short-term effects, lasting 4–6 hours. Stimulants should be initiated at a low dosage, and the dosage should be increased according to response and adverse effects within the recommended dosage range. These agents are given after meals to reduce the likelihood of appetite suppression. Both stimulant and nonstimulant drugs are available in slow- or extended-release formulations.

Early adverse effects include appetite suppression, weight loss, irritability, abdominal pain, and insomnia. Mild dysphoria and social withdrawal could occur at higher dosages in some patients. Any decrease in expected weight gain is small and likely insignificant. Treatment with stimulants is not associated with later risk for substance use disorders.

Parents can benefit from learning basic behavioral management skills, such as the value of positive reinforcement and firm, nonpunitive limit setting, as well as methods for reducing stimulation, thereby diminishing distractibility and inattentiveness.

Specific Learning Disorder

Specific learning disorder is characterized by an inability to achieve in a designated area of learning at a level consistent with the person's overall intellectual functioning. The essential feature is a persistent problem in acquiring or learning academic skills as quickly or as accurately as peers during the years of formal schooling (i.e., the developmental period). Academic skills will be well below the average range for the individual's age. Reading disorders often are called *dyslexia*. A commonly used term for mathematic disorders is *dyscalculia*. Specific learning disorder affects approximately 5%–15% of school-age children; it is two to three times more common in boys than in girls.

Children or teenagers will need remedial instruction to bolster their academic skills, as well as instruction in developing "attack" skills that will assist them in learning strategies to compensate for the neural deficits that underlie their condition. Steady, sympathetic educational support will enable most children with these deficits to develop acceptable skills in reading, writing, and arithmetic.

Motor Disorders

Developmental Coordination Disorder

The essential feature of developmental coordination disorder is a marked impairment in acquisition of skills requiring motor coordination. Children with the disorder usually are seen as physically awkward by their parents and peers. Younger children could display delays and clumsiness in achieving developmental motor milestones such as crawling, sitting, and walking, while older children might display difficulties with motor aspects of assembling puzzles or building models or participating in sports activities. Developmental coordination disorder must be distinguished from other medical conditions that could produce coordination problems, such as cerebral palsy, muscular dystrophy, visual impairment, or an intellectual developmental disorder.

Stereotypic Movement Disorder

Stereotypic movement disorder is characterized by repetitive, seemingly driven, and apparently purposeless motor behaviors that interfere with social, academic, and other activities or result in self-injury. Typical movements can include hand waving, rocking, playing with hands, fiddling with fingers, twirling objects, head banging, and self-biting. This disorder has an onset in early childhood and needs to be distinguished from neurological conditions and from other neurodevelopmental or mental disorders (e.g., Tourette's disorder).

Tic Disorders

People with tic disorders have stereotypical but nonrhythmic "jerky" movements and vocalizations called *tics*. The best known are Tourette's disorder, persistent (chronic) motor or vocal tic disorder, and provisional tic disorder.

Tourette's Disorder

Tourette's disorder involves the production of motor and vocal tics. The vocal tics can be somewhat socially offensive, such as making loud grunting or barking noises or shouting words. The patient is aware that he or she is producing the vocal tics and is able to exert a mild degree of control over them, but ultimately has to submit to them. Motor tics occurring in Tourette's disorder are often odd or offensive behaviors, such as tongue protrusion, sniffing, hopping, squatting, blinking, or nodding. Because most of the general public is unaware of the nature of Tourette's disorder, the behavior is seen as inappropriate or bizarre and usually causes embarrassment to the patient. The tics tend to worsen when the individual is anxious, excited, or fatigued. The DSM-5 criteria for Tourette's disorder are shown in Box 3–4.

Box 3–4.   DSM-5 Criteria for Tourette's Disorder

Note: A tic is a sudden, rapid, recurrent, nonrhythmic motor movement or vocalization.

A. Both multiple motor and one or more vocal tics have been present at some time during the illness, although not necessarily concurrently.
B. The tics may wax and wane in frequency but have persisted for more than 1 year since first tic onset.
C. Onset is before age 18 years.
D. The disturbance is not attributable to the physiological effects of a substance (e.g., cocaine) or another medical condition (e.g., Huntington's disease, postviral encephalitis).

The disorder affects 3–8 schoolchildren per 1,000. Tics themselves are common in childhood but tend to be transient. Tourette's disorder is more common in boys than in girls, with a ratio of approximately 3:1. Tics often begin between ages 4 and 6 years, with motor tics generally preceding the appearance of vocal tics. Tic severity tends to peak between ages 10 and 12. People often have fewer symptoms as they age, although a small percentage will have persistently severe or worsening symptoms in adulthood.

Tourette's disorder is highly familial and comorbid with obsessive-compulsive disorder. Clinically, tics and compulsions have a superficial resemblance, suggesting that these symptoms might lie along a continuum.

Some children with Tourette's disorder experience onset of symptoms after infection with group A beta-hemolytic *Streptococcus*. Streptococcal infections are a well-known cause of Sydenham's chorea, and it now appears that Tourette's disorder is a related condition. This group of syndromes is referred to as a *pediatric autoimmune neuropsychiatric disorder associated with streptococcal infections* (PANDAS).

Evaluation should include a comprehensive neurological evaluation to rule out other possible causes of the tics. Examine the patient for the stigmata of Wilson's disease, and obtain a family history to evaluate the possibility of Huntington's disease. Also evaluate the patient for comorbid ADHD and learning disorders, as well as mood and anxiety disorders.

Tourette's disorder also must be differentiated from persistent (chronic) motor or vocal tic disorder, which is characterized by the presence of motor tics or vocal tics but not both. Other clinical features are the same for both conditions, including onset before age 18 years. The diagnosis of a persistent tic disorder cannot be made if the individual has ever had symptoms that met the criteria for Tourette's disorder.

Treatment is often started with low dosages of alpha-adrenergic drugs (e.g., clonidine, 0.2–0.3 mg/day; guanfacine, 1.5–4 mg/day). Antipsychotics usually are prescribed if adrenergic medications are ineffective. Pimozide is FDA approved to treat Tourette's disorder, but second-generation antipsychotics (e.g., risperidone, 1–3 mg/day; ziprasidone, 20–40 mg/day) often are better tolerated. It is important to educate the family about the disorder and to assist them in providing psychological support to the patient.

Other "Adult" Disorders Frequently Seen in Children

Schizophrenia often has its onset during adolescence, but in rare instances the onset is during childhood. Schizophrenia in adolescents typically begins insidiously, with apathy, a change in personal hygiene, and withdrawal. The major challenge in assessing childhood schizophrenia involves determining the difference between normal childhood fantasies and frank delusions and hallucinations. In addition, the symptoms of disorganization of speech and behavior must be distinguished from any abnormalities of speech and behavior that are simply due to developmental slowness or intellectual disability.

Up to 5% of children and 8% of adolescents have symptoms that meet the diagnostic criteria for major depression. The patient with major depression may present initially with physical complaints rather than the psychological complaint of depression. In young children, the complaints may be abdominal pain, nightmares, or trouble sleeping. In teenagers, complaints of fatigue, insomnia or hypersomnia, headache, or tension are common. Depression also may present initially with disruptive behavior such as that seen in oppositional defiant disorder or conduct disorder. A combination of medication and psychotherapy might provide the best chance for recovery. Fluoxetine and escitalopram are FDA-approved for the treatment of pediatric depression and should be used as first-line medications.

In 2003, the FDA issued a black box warning about the risk of increased suicidal behavior in children, adolescents, and young adults (<25 years) taking antidepressants and advised "close supervision" of such patients. There is some evidence that the warning may have led to an increase in suicidal behaviors, because many cases of depression have gone untreated.

Bipolar disorder presenting with mania is also becoming increasingly recognized in children and adolescents. This has led to some controversy, because many of its symptoms overlap with those of ADHD and other disruptive behavior disorders. In mania, the child will be overly happy, giddy, or euphoric. Sometimes the child will just be irritable. Bipolar disorder in children is generally treated with the same medications used in adults, though usually at lower doses. Asenapine, a second-generation antipsychotic, is FDA-approved in the treatment of pediatric bipolar I disorder.

Clinical Points for Neurodevelopmental (Child) Disorders

- When assessing children and adolescents, be imaginative and meet each patient on his or her own terms.

  - Problem-solving and motor skills can be evaluated by playing games.

- Dolls and toys can be used with young children to create pretend situations that will provide insight about personal and social interactions.
- Normal maturational levels are highly variable in children and adolescents.
- Children and adolescents often do not have a level of cognitive development suitable for the insight-oriented and introspective approaches used with adults.
- Establishing rapport with adolescents is difficult but might be crucial to creating a therapeutic alliance.
  - The therapist should find out what the patient is interested in and relate to him or her through these interests.
- Do not preach or judge.
- The basic maturational task of adolescents is to disengage themselves from their parents, become independent, and define their own identities; reliance on peers is an important crutch for adolescents in this transitional period.
- Remain neutral and try not to criticize either parents or peers.
- The adolescent's first reaction might be to see the therapist as a parent. Try to use this to therapeutic advantage, or at least try to prevent it from being a therapeutic handicap.
- Be aware of the pervasiveness of comorbidity in childhood and adolescent disorders.

Further Reading

American Association on Intellectual and Developmental Disabilities: Intellectual Disability: Definition, Classification, and Systems of Support, 11th Edition. Washington, DC, American Association on Intellectual and Developmental Disabilities, 2010

Berninger VW, May MO: Evidence-based diagnosis and treatment for specific learning disabilities involving impairments in written and/or oral language. J Learn Disabil 44(2):167–183, 2011

Cepeda C: Clinical Manual for the Psychiatric Interview of Children and Adolescents. Washington, DC, American Psychiatric Publishing, 2009

Doyle CA, McDougle CJ: Pharmacologic treatments for the behavioral symptoms associated with autism spectrum disorders across the lifespan. Dialogues Clin Neurosci 14(3):263–279, 2012

Dulcan M (ed): Dulcan's Textbook of Child and Adolescent Psychiatry, 2nd Edition. Arlington, VA, American Psychiatric Association Publishing, 2016

Ghaziuddin M: Asperger disorder in the DSM-V: sacrificing utility for validity. J Am Acad Child Adolesc Psychiatry 50(2):192–193, 2011

Hollander E, Kalevzon A, Coyle JT (eds): Textbook of Autism Spectrum Disorders. Washington, DC, American Psychiatric Publishing, 2011

McNaught KS, Mink JW: Advances in understanding and treatment of Tourette syndrome. Nat Rev Neurol 7(12):667–676, 2011

Quinn PD, Chang Z, Hur K, et al: ADHD medication and substance-related problems. Am J Psychiatry 174(9):877–885, 2017

Vismara LA, Rogers SJ: Behavioral treatments in autism spectrum disorder: what do we know? Annu Rev Clin Psychol 6:447–468, 2010

Chapter 4

Schizophrenia Spectrum and Other Psychotic Disorders

DSM-5 recognizes a spectrum of psychotic disorders related to schizophrenia. All are united by the presence of disturbance in one of the five domains of psychopathology: delusions, hallucinations, disorganized thinking, grossly disorganized/catatonic behavior, and negative symptoms. The DSM-5 schizophrenia spectrum and other psychotic disorders are listed in Table 4–1.

Delusional Disorder

The core feature of delusional disorder is the presence of a well-systematized delusion in the absence of obviously odd or bizarre behavior. The person might seem relatively normal other than for the immediate impact of the delusion. If hallucinations are present, they are not prominent and are related to the theme of the delusion. The DSM-5 diagnostic criteria for delusional disorder are shown in Box 4–1.

Box 4–1.   DSM-5 Criteria for Delusional Disorder

A. The presence of one (or more) delusions with a duration of 1 month or longer.

B. Criterion A for schizophrenia has never been met.
   Note: Hallucinations, if present, are not prominent and are related to the delusional theme (e.g., the sensation of being infested with insects associated with delusions of infestation).

C. Apart from the impact of the delusion(s) or its ramifications, functioning is not markedly impaired, and behavior is not obviously bizarre or odd.

D. If manic or major depressive episodes have occurred, these have been brief relative to the duration of the delusional periods.

E. The disturbance is not attributable to the physiological effects of a substance or another medical condition and is not better explained by another mental disorder, such as body dysmorphic disorder or obsessive-compulsive disorder.

The clinician should specify one of the following subtypes:

- **Erotomanic type:** The central theme of the delusion is that another person is in love with the individual.
- **Grandiose type:** The central theme of the delusion is the conviction of having some great (but unrecognized) talent or insight or having made some important discovery.
- **Jealous type:** The central theme of the individual's delusion is that his or her spouse or lover is unfaithful.
- **Persecutory type:** The central theme of the delusion involves the individual's belief that he or she is being conspired against, cheated, spied on, followed, poisoned or drugged, maliciously maligned, harassed, or obstructed in the pursuit of long-term goals.
- **Somatic type:** The central theme of the delusion involves bodily functions or sensations.
- **Mixed type:** No one delusional theme predominates.
- **Unspecified type:** The dominant delusional belief cannot be clearly determined or is not described in the specific types (e.g., referential delusions without a prominent persecutory or grandiose component).

The clinician also can specify if the content of delusions is bizarre ("with bizarre content"). Delusional disorder has a prevalence of about 0.2% in the general population. There are no major gender differences, and the disorder is observed in middle to late adult life. Delusional disorder has a significant familial relationship with schizophrenia and schizotypal personality disorder.

People with delusional disorder tend to be socially isolated and chronically suspicious. Those with persecutory or jealous delusions sometimes can become angry and hostile, emotions that can lead to violent outbursts. The jealous subtype appears to be the most common.

The primary differential diagnosis involves distinguishing delusional disorder from mood disorders, schizophrenia, paranoid personality disorder, and body dysmorphic disorder.

Delusional disorder usually is treated with antipsychotics, but response often is poor. Antipsychotics might help relieve

TABLE 4–1. DSM-5 schizophrenia spectrum and other psychotic disorders

Schizotypal personality disorder[a]

Delusional disorder

Brief psychotic disorder

Schizophreniform disorder

Schizophrenia

Schizoaffective disorder

Substance/medication-induced psychotic disorder

Psychotic disorder due to another medical condition

Catatonia associated with another mental disorder (catatonia specifier)

Catatonic disorder due to another medical condition

[a]See Chapter 17, "Personality Disorders."

agitation and anxiety but leave the core delusion intact. Any antipsychotic can be used, but second-generation antipsychotics (SGAs) tend to be better tolerated. The somatic type of delusional disorder might respond better to pimozide. Selective serotonin reuptake inhibitors (SSRIs) also have been reported to help reduce delusional beliefs in some patients.

Clinical Points for Delusional Disorder

- Because a patient with delusional disorder is suspicious, it may be very difficult to establish a therapeutic relationship.

    - Building a relationship will take time and patience.

    - Neither condemn nor collude in the delusional beliefs of the patient.

    - Assure the patient of complete confidentiality.

- Once rapport is established, the patient's delusional beliefs can be gently challenged by pointing out how they interfere with his or her functioning.

    - Tact and skill are needed to convince the patient to accept treatment.

- A patient with delusional disorder may be more accepting of medication if it is described as a treatment for anxiety, dysphoria, and stress that may result from or accompany his or her delusions.

  - Antipsychotic medication should be tried, although results are unpredictable; SGAs will be better tolerated.

  - Patients with the somatic subtype might respond better to pimozide.

Brief Psychotic Disorder

Patients with a brief psychotic disorder have psychotic symptoms that last at least 1 day but less than 1 month, with gradual recovery. Psychotic mood disorders, schizophrenia, and the effects of drugs or medical conditions have been ruled out as the cause of the symptoms. Signs and symptoms are similar to those seen in schizophrenia, including hallucinations, delusions, and disorganized speech or grossly disorganized behavior. There are four specifiers: 1) with marked stressor(s), 2) without marked stressor(s), 3) with postpartum onset, and 4) with catatonia.

The prevalence of brief psychotic disorder may be as high as 9% of new-onset psychoses, and the disorder is twice as common among women. Brief psychotic disorder is thought to occur more commonly in lower-income groups and among those with personality disorders, especially borderline and schizotypal types. Patients with brief psychotic disorder of postpartum onset generally develop symptoms during pregnancy or within 4 weeks after delivery. Symptoms tend to arise in otherwise psychiatrically healthy individuals and resolve within 2–3 months.

Antipsychotics can be helpful early on, especially when the patient is highly agitated or experiencing great emotional turmoil. Hospitalization might be necessary for the safety of the patient or others.

Schizophreniform Disorder

Schizophreniform disorder is a diagnosis for patients who present with symptoms typical of schizophrenia but have been ill for less than 6 months. In DSM-5, the definition requires that 1) the patient have psychotic symptoms characteristic of schizophrenia, such as hallucinations, delusions, or disorganized speech; 2) the symptoms not be due to the physiological effects of a substance, or a medication or another medical condition; 3) schizoaffective disorder and mood disorder with psychotic features have been ruled out; and 4) the duration is at least 1 month but less than 6 months.

The diagnosis changes to schizophrenia if the condition persists past 6 months, even if only residual symptoms (e.g., blunted affect) remain. The diagnosis appears to identify a widely varying group of patients, most of whom eventually develop schizophrenia, a mood disorder, or schizoaffective disorder. Treatment recommendations are the same as for schizophrenia.

Schizophrenia

In DSM-5, *schizophrenia* is defined by a group of characteristic symptoms, such as hallucinations, delusions, or negative symptoms (i.e., affective flattening, alogia, avolition); deterioration in social, occupational, or interpersonal relationships; and continuous signs of the disturbance for at least 6 months. The DSM-5 diagnostic criteria for schizophrenia are shown in Box 4–2.

Box 4–2. DSM-5 Criteria for Schizophrenia

A. Two (or more) of the following, each present for a significant portion of time during a 1-month period (or less if successfully treated). At least one of these must be (1), (2), or (3):

1. Delusions.
2. Hallucinations.
3. Disorganized speech (e.g., frequent derailment or incoherence).
4. Grossly disorganized or catatonic behavior.
5. Negative symptoms (i.e., diminished emotional expression or avolition).

B. For a significant portion of the time since the onset of the disturbance, level of functioning in one or more major areas, such as work, interpersonal relations, or self-care, is markedly below the level achieved prior to the onset (or when the onset is in childhood or adolescence, there is failure to achieve expected level of interpersonal, academic, or occupational functioning).

C. Continuous signs of the disturbance persist for at least 6 months. This 6-month period must include at least 1 month of symptoms (or less if successfully treated) that meet Criterion A (i.e., active-phase symptoms) and may include periods of prodromal or residual symptoms. During these prodromal or residual periods, the signs of the disturbance may be manifested by only negative symptoms or by two or more symptoms listed in Criterion A present in an attenuated form (e.g., odd beliefs, unusual perceptual experiences).

D. Schizoaffective disorder and depressive or bipolar disorder with psychotic features have been ruled out because either 1) no major depressive or manic episodes have occurred concurrently with the active-phase symptoms, or 2) if mood episodes have occurred during active-phase symptoms, they have been present for a minority of the total duration of the active and residual periods of the illness.

E. The disturbance is not attributable to the physiological effects of a substance (e.g., a drug of abuse, a medication) or another medical condition.

F. If there is a history of autism spectrum disorder or a communication disorder of childhood onset, the additional diagnosis of schizophrenia is made only if prominent delusions or hallucinations, in addition to the other required symptoms of schizophrenia, are also present for at least 1 month (or less if successfully treated).

Epidemiology

The prevalence of schizophrenia is approximately 0.5%–1%. The common age at onset is 18–25 years for men and 21–30 years for women. Patients with schizophrenia often do not marry and are less likely to have children than others.

Clinical Findings

Three groups of symptoms have been described:

- *Psychoticism:* positive symptoms (i.e., symptoms characterized by the presence of something that should be absent, such as hearing voices)
- *Negative dimension:* negative symptoms (i.e., symptoms characterized by the absence of something that should be present, such as avolition [lack of motivation])

- *Disorganization dimension:* disorganized speech and behavior and inappropriate affect

Psychoticism

Hallucinations and delusions are the two classic "psychotic" symptoms that reflect a patient's confusion about the loss of boundaries between himself or herself and the external world. *Hallucinations* are perceptions experienced without an external stimulus to the sense organs.

- *Auditory hallucinations* are the most frequent and typically are experienced as speech ("voices"). The voices may be mumbled or heard clearly, and they may be heard as words, phrases, or sentences.
- *Visual hallucinations* may be simple or complex and include flashes of light, persons, animals, or objects.
- *Olfactory and gustatory hallucinations* often are experienced together, especially as unpleasant tastes or odors.
- *Tactile hallucinations* might be experienced as sensations of being touched or pricked or as electrical sensations.
- *Delusions* are fixed false beliefs that are untrue as well as contrary to a person's educational and cultural background. Delusions have varied content, as shown in Table 4–2.

Negative Dimension

In DSM-5, two negative symptoms are characteristic of schizophrenia: diminished emotional expression and avolition. Other negative symptoms common in schizophrenia are alogia and anhedonia. These symptoms are described below.

- *Diminished emotional expression (affective flattening or blunting)* is a reduced intensity of emotional expression and response. It is manifested by unchanging facial expression, decreased spontaneous movements, poverty of expressive gestures, poor eye contact, lack of voice inflections, and slowed speech.
- *Avolition* is a loss of the ability to initiate goal-directed behavior and carry it through to completion. Patients seem inert and unmotivated.
- *Alogia* is characterized by a diminution in the amount of spontaneous speech or a tendency to produce speech that is empty or impoverished in content when the amount is adequate.

TABLE 4–2. Focus of content in delusions

Delusions	Foci of preoccupation
Grandiose	Possessing wealth or great beauty or having special abilities; having influential friends; being an important historical figure
Nihilistic	Believing that one is dead or dying; believing that one does not exist or that the world does not exist
Persecutory	Being persecuted by friends, neighbors, or a spouse; being followed, monitored, or spied on by the government or other important organizations
Somatic	Believing that one's organs have stopped functioning (e.g., that the heart is no longer beating) or are rotting away; believing that the nose or another body part is terribly misshapen or disfigured
Sexual	Believing that one's sexual behavior is commonly known; that one is a prostitute, pedophile, or rapist; that masturbation has led to illness or insanity
Religious	Believing that one has sinned against God or that one has a special relationship to God or some other deity; that one has a special religious mission; that one is the Devil or is condemned to Hell

- *Anhedonia* is the inability to experience pleasure. Patients may describe themselves as feeling emotionally empty and unable to enjoy activities that previously gave them pleasure, such as playing sports or visiting with family or friends.

Disorganization Dimension

The *disorganization dimension* refers to disorganized speech, disorganized or bizarre behavior, and inappropriate affect. Disorganized speech, or *thought disorder*, involves abnormalities in thought and communication that include loose associations, poverty of speech, poverty of content of speech, and tangential replies. Types of thought disorders are described in Chapter 2. With *inappropriate affect*, patients might smile inappropriately when speaking of neutral or sad topics, or may giggle for no apparent reason.

Many patients with schizophrenia also have different types of disorganized motor and social behavior (also described in Chapter 2), including the following:

- *Catatonic stupor:* The patient is immobile, mute, and unresponsive, yet fully conscious.
- *Catatonic excitement:* The patient has uncontrolled and aimless motor activity. Patients sometimes assume bizarre or uncomfortable postures (e.g., squatting) and maintain them for long periods.
- *Stereotypy:* The patient has a repeated but non-goal-directed movement, such as back-and-forth rocking.
- *Mannerisms:* The patient exhibits goal-directed activities that are either odd in appearance or out of context, such as grimacing.
- *Echopraxia:* The patient imitates movements and gestures of another person.
- *Automatic obedience:* The patient carries out simple commands in a robot-like fashion.
- *Negativism:* The patient refuses to cooperate with simple requests for no apparent reason.

Most patients with schizophrenia lack insight and do not believe they are ill. They often reject the idea that they need treatment. Comorbid substance abuse is very common. Patients who abuse substances tend to be young, male, and poorly adherent with treatment.

Course of Illness

About one-third of patients first diagnosed with schizophrenia will have a relatively good outcome, with minimal symptoms and mild impairments in cognition and social functioning; one-third will have a poor outcome, with persisting psychotic symptoms, prominent negative symptoms, and significant psychosocial impairment; and one-third will have an outcome somewhere in the middle.

Typical stages of schizophrenia are outlined in Table 4–3. Features associated with good outcome include female gender, acute (rather than insidious) onset, good premorbid functioning, and high intelligence.

Differential Diagnosis

The major differential diagnosis involves separating schizophrenia from schizoaffective disorder, a mood disorder, delusional disorder, and personality disorders. A thorough history will help to rule out cases of psychosis due to substances of abuse (e.g., stimulants, hallucinogens, phencyclidine); certain

TABLE 4–3. Typical stages of schizophrenia

Stage	Features
Prodromal phase	Insidious onset occurs over months or years; subtle behavior changes include social withdrawal, work impairment, blunting of emotion, avolition, and odd ideas and behavior.
Active phase	Psychotic symptoms, including hallucinations, delusions, or disorganized speech and behavior, develop. These symptoms eventually lead to medical intervention.
Residual phase	Active-phase symptoms are absent or no longer prominent. There often is role impairment, negative symptoms, or attenuated positive symptoms. Acute-phase symptoms may reemerge during the residual phase ("acute exacerbation").

medications (e.g., corticosteroids, anticholinergics, levodopa); infections; metabolic and endocrine disorders; tumors and mass lesions; and temporal lobe epilepsy. The medical workup should include a complete blood count, urinalysis, liver enzymes, serum creatinine, blood urea nitrogen, thyroid function tests, and serologic tests for evidence of an infection with syphilis or HIV. Magnetic resonance imaging (MRI) can be helpful for some patients to rule out focal brain disorder (e.g., tumors, strokes) in new-onset cases. (See Table 4–4 for the differential diagnosis of schizophrenia.)

Etiology and Pathophysiology

Schizophrenia is best considered a "multiple-hit" illness similar to cancer, diabetes, and cardiovascular disease. Individuals might carry a genetic predisposition, but this vulnerability is not "released" unless other factors also intervene.

Genetics

Schizophrenia is highly heritable. Family studies have shown that siblings of schizophrenia patients have approximately a 10% chance of developing schizophrenia, whereas children who have one parent with schizophrenia have a 5%–6% chance. Studies are underway to identify vulnerability genes.

TABLE 4–4. Differential diagnosis of schizophrenia

Psychiatric illness	Other medical illness
Bipolar disorder	Temporal lobe epilepsy
Major depression	Tumor, stroke, brain trauma
Schizoaffective disorder	Endocrine/metabolic disorders (e.g., porphyria)
Brief psychotic disorder	
Schizophreniform disorder	Vitamin deficiency (e.g., B_{12})
Delusional disorder	Infectious disease (e.g., neurosyphilis)
Panic disorder	
Depersonalization disorder	Autoimmune disorder (e.g., systemic lupus erythematosus)
Obsessive-compulsive disorder	Toxic illness (e.g., heavy metal poisoning)
Personality disorders	
	Drugs
	Stimulants (e.g., amphetamine, cocaine)
	Hallucinogens
	Anticholinergics (e.g., belladonna alkaloids)
	Alcohol withdrawal
	Barbiturate withdrawal

Imaging Studies

Cerebral ventricular enlargement, sulcal enlargement, and cerebellar atrophy have been observed in schizophrenia patients. Ventricular enlargement is associated with poor premorbid functioning, negative symptoms, poor response to treatment, and cognitive impairment. MRI studies have shown decreased frontal lobe size. Longitudinal studies show that progressive tissue loss occurs over time in some patients, but the mechanism remains unknown. Several studies have found decreased thalamus size in patients with schizophrenia.

Functional Neuroimaging

Patients with schizophrenia have a relative "hypofrontality" that is associated with prominent negative symptoms.

Neurodevelopmental Influences

Patients with schizophrenia are more likely than control subjects to have a history of birth injury and perinatal complications that could result in a subtle brain injury, therefore setting the stage for the development of schizophrenia.

Neurochemistry and Neuropharmacology

The "dopamine hypothesis" suggests that symptoms of schizophrenia arise from a functional hyperactivity in the dopamine system in limbic regions and a functional hypoactivity in frontal regions. The efficacy of many antipsychotic drugs used to treat schizophrenia is highly correlated with their ability to block dopamine (D_2) receptors. The newer SGAs were developed to have a broader pharmacological profile and also block serotonin type 2 (5-HT_2) receptors, suggesting a role for serotonin in the pathophysiology of schizophrenia. Glutamate also is being studied as a possible contributor to development of schizophrenia. One hypothesis is that there is a hypofunction in the N-methyl-D-aspartate receptors within the glutamate system.

Clinical Management

Antipsychotic medication is the mainstay of treatment. The uses, dosages, mechanisms of action, metabolism, and adverse effects of these agents are described in Chapter 21.

Treatment of Acute Psychosis

High-potency first-generation antipsychotics (FGAs) and SGAs are first-line treatments. SGAs generally are better tolerated because they are less likely to cause extrapyramidal side effects, but they can cause weight gain, glucose intolerance, and lipid dysregulation. Clozapine is a second-line choice because it can in rare cases cause agranulocytosis. Nonetheless, it is associated with reduced suicidal behavior and might be more effective than the other antipsychotics.

Maintenance Therapy

Sustained control of psychotic symptoms is the goal of maintenance treatment. At least 1–2 years of treatment with antipsychotics are recommended after the initial episode because of the high risk of relapse. At least 5 years of treatment for multiple episodes are recommended because a high risk of relapse remains. Long-acting injectable antipsychotics are helpful in patients who lack insight or are chronically non-compliant.

Adjunctive Treatments

Many patients benefit from benzodiazepines when anxiety is prominent. Lithium, valproate, and carbamazepine can be used to reduce impulsive and aggressive behaviors, hyperactivity, or mood swings, although their effectiveness in patients with schizophrenia has not been fully determined and their use is off-label. Antidepressants sometimes are used to treat depression in schizophrenia patients and appear effective. Electroconvulsive therapy sometimes is used, particularly to treat concurrent depression or catatonic symptoms.

Psychosocial Interventions

Reserve hospitalization for patients who pose a danger to themselves or others; are unable to properly care for themselves (e.g., refuse food or fluids); or require special medical observation, tests, or treatments. Some patients may benefit from the structure of a partial hospitalization program or day hospital.

Other Approaches

- *Assertive community treatment* (ACT) programs employ careful monitoring of patients through mobile mental health teams and individually tailored programming. These programs reduce hospital admission rates and improve the patient's quality of life.
- *Family therapy*, combined with antipsychotic medication, has been shown to reduce relapse rates in patients with schizophrenia.
- *Cognitive rehabilitation* involves the remediation of abnormal thought processes known to occur in schizophrenia, using methods pioneered in the treatment of brain-injured persons.
- *Social skills training* (SST) aims to help patients develop more appropriate social behavior.
- *Psychosocial rehabilitation* serves to integrate the patient back into his or her community rather than segregating the pa-

tient in a separate facility. This could involve patient club-
houses to encourage socialization.

- *Vocational rehabilitation* aims to help the patient obtain sup-
ported employment, competitive work in integrated settings, and more formal job training programs.

Clinical Points for Schizophrenia

- Treat psychotic symptoms aggressively with medication.

  - High-potency FGAs and SGAs are considered first-line
  therapy because they are effective and well tolerated.

  - Intramuscular medication is useful in cases of patient
  noncompliance or for patients who prefer the convenience of bimonthly or monthly injections.

- Engage the patient in an empathic relationship.

  - This task may at times be challenging because some
  patients are unemotional, aloof, and withdrawn.

  - The clinician should be practical and help the patient
  with problems that matter to him or her, such as finding
  adequate housing.

- Help the patient find a daily routine that he or she can manage, to improve socialization and reduce boredom.

  - Partial hospitalization or day treatment programs are
  available in many areas.

  - Sheltered workshops that provide simple, repetitive
  chores may be helpful.

- Develop a close working relationship with local social services.

  - Patients with schizophrenia tend to be poor and disabled;
  finding adequate housing and food requires the skills of
  a social worker.

  - Help the patient obtain disability benefits.

- Family therapy is important for the patient who lives at home
or who still has close family ties.

  - As a result of the illness, many patients will have broken
  their family ties.

- Families desperately need education about schizophrenia.

- Help family members find a support group through referral to a local chapter of the National Alliance on Mental Illness (NAMI).

Schizoaffective Disorder

The hallmark of schizoaffective disorder is the presence of either a depressive or manic episode concurrent with symptoms characteristic of schizophrenia, such as delusions, hallucinations, or disorganized speech. (See Box 4–3 for the DSM-5 diagnostic criteria for schizoaffective disorder.) There are two subtypes: the *bipolar type*, marked by a current or previous manic syndrome, and the *depressive type*, marked by the absence of any manic syndromes.

Box 4–3.   DSM-5 Criteria for Schizoaffective Disorder

A. An uninterrupted period of illness during which there is a major mood episode (major depressive or manic) concurrent with Criterion A of schizophrenia.
   Note: The major depressive episode must include Criterion A1: Depressed mood.
B. Delusions or hallucinations for 2 or more weeks in the absence of a major mood episode (depressive or manic) during the lifetime duration of the illness.
C. Symptoms that meet criteria for a major mood episode are present for the majority of the total duration of the active and residual portions of the illness.
D. The disturbance is not attributable to the effects of a substance (e.g., a drug of abuse, a medication) or another medical condition.

Schizoaffective disorder has an estimated prevalence of less than 1% and occurs more often in women. The signs and symptoms of schizoaffective disorder include those seen in schizophrenia and mood disorders. The symptoms might present together or in an alternating fashion, and psychotic symptoms may be mood congruent or mood incongruent. The course of schizoaffective disorder is variable but represents a middle ground between that of schizophrenia and mood disorders.

The differential diagnosis for schizoaffective disorder consists primarily of schizophrenia, the mood disorders, and disorders induced by medical conditions or drugs of abuse.

Treatment should target mood and psychotic symptoms. The SGA paliperidone is FDA-approved to treat schizoaffective disorder. Some patients may benefit from adding a mood stabilizer (e.g., lithium, valproate) or an antidepressant. Patients not responding to medication may respond to electroconvulsive therapy.

Further Reading

Cascade E, Kalali AH, Buckley P: Treatment of schizoaffective disorder. Psychiatry (Edgmont) 6(3):15–17, 2009

Coldwell CM, Bender WS: The effectiveness of assertive community treatment for homeless populations with severe mental illness: a meta-analysis. Am J Psychiatry 164(3):393–399, 2007

Essock SM, Covell NH, Davis SM, et al: Effectiveness of switching antipsychotic medications. Am J Psychiatry 163(12):2090–2095, 2006

Goff DC, Falkai P, Fleischhacker WW, et al: The long-term effects of antipsychotic medication on clinical course of schizophrenia. Am J Psychiatry 174(9):840–849, 2017

Green AI, Drake RE, Brunette MF, Noordsy DL: Schizophrenia and co-occurring substance use disorder. Am J Psychiatry 164(3):402–408, 2007

Huxley NA, Rendall M, Sederer L: Psychosocial treatments in schizophrenia: a review of the past 20 years. J Nerv Ment Dis 188(4):187–201, 2000

Kane JM: New-onset schizophrenia: pharmacologic treatment. Focus 6:167–171, 2008

Lauriello J, Pallanti S (eds): Clinical Manual for Treatment of Schizophrenia. Washington, DC, American Psychiatric Publishing, 2012

Lieberman JA, Stroup TS, Perkins DO (eds): Essentials of Schizophrenia. Washington, DC, American Psychiatric Publishing, 2012

Stroup TS, Lieberman JA, McEvoy JP, et al; CATIE Investigators: Effectiveness of olanzapine, quetiapine, and risperidone in patients with chronic schizophrenia after discontinuing perphenazine: a CATIE study. Am J Psychiatry 164(3):415–427, 2007

Chapter 5

Mood Disorders

Mood disorders have a high prevalence, high morbidity, and high mortality. Among people ages 15–45 years, depression accounts for an astonishing 10.3% of all health care costs worldwide. Bipolar disorder ranks sixth among the world's most disabling illnesses. All physicians who have direct personal contact with patients should learn the fundamentals of diagnosing and treating mood disorders. In DSM-5, bipolar and related disorders and depressive disorders are in separate chapters. For convenience, they are combined in this chapter.

Diagnosis

Bipolar and Related Disorders

This diagnostic class recognizes disorders characterized by marked swings in mood, activity, and behavior. The categorization includes bipolar I and bipolar II disorder, cyclothymic disorder, substance/medication-induced bipolar and related disorder, and bipolar and related disorder due to another medical condition (Table 5–1).

Manic Episode

DSM-5 criteria for a manic episode require the presence of an abnormally elevated, expansive, or irritable mood lasting at least 1 week plus at least three (or four if the mood is irritable) of seven characteristic symptoms (Box 5–1). The criteria are similar to those used to define depression in that the mood disturbance must be sufficiently severe to cause marked impairment or require hospitalization.

Box 5–1.   DSM-5 Criteria for Manic Episode

A. A distinct period of abnormally and persistently elevated, expansive, or irritable mood and abnormally and persistently increased activity or energy, lasting at least 1 week and present most of the day, nearly every day (or any duration if hospitalization is necessary).

B. During the period of mood disturbance and increased energy or activity, three (or more) of the following symptoms (four if the mood is only irritable) are present to a significant degree and represent a noticeable change from usual behavior:

   1. Inflated self-esteem or grandiosity.
   2. Decreased need for sleep (e.g., feels rested after only 3 hours of sleep).
   3. More talkative than usual or pressure to keep talking.
   4. Flight of ideas or subjective experience that thoughts are racing.
   5. Distractibility (i.e., attention too easily drawn to unimportant or irrelevant external stimuli), as reported or observed.
   6. Increase in goal-directed activity (either socially, at work or school, or sexually) or psychomotor agitation (i.e., purposeless non-goal-directed activity).
   7. Excessive involvement in activities that have a high potential for painful consequences (e.g., engaging in unrestrained buying sprees, sexual indiscretions, or foolish business investments).

C. The mood disturbance is sufficiently severe to cause marked impairment in social or occupational functioning or to necessitate hospitalization to prevent harm to self or others, or there are psychotic features.

D. The episode is not attributable to the physiological effects of a substance (e.g., a drug of abuse, a medication, other treatment) or another medical condition.

   Note: A full manic episode that emerges during antidepressant treatment (e.g., medication, electroconvulsive therapy) but persists at a fully syndromal level beyond the physiological effect of that treatment is sufficient evidence for a manic episode and, therefore, a bipolar I diagnosis.

Note: Criteria A–D constitute a manic episode. At least one lifetime manic episode is required for the diagnosis of bipolar I disorder.

TABLE 5–1. DSM-5 bipolar and related disorders

Bipolar I disorder

Bipolar II disorder

Cyclothymic disorder

Substance/medication-induced bipolar and related disorder

Bipolar and related disorder due to another medical condition

Bipolar I disorder is defined by the occurrence of at least one manic or mixed episode. Typically, bipolar I disorder is characterized by recurrent episodes of mania and depression, which can be separated by months or years.

Clinical findings. The patient's mood typically is cheerful, enthusiastic, and expansive. The cheerfulness often has an infectious quality, making interviewing an enjoyable and sometimes amusing experience. Other times, however, the patient's mood is simply irritable, particularly if the person feels thwarted, and these irritable manic patients can be quite difficult to manage. Other symptoms include the following:

- Manic patients might believe that they have *special abilities* or powers. Inflated self-esteem and grandiosity could reach delusional proportions.
- Patients could experience *increased activity or energy*. These individuals might be physically restless and unable to sit still. The increased activity level often is accompanied by poor judgment.
- Patients with mania tend to *overextend themselves* in ways that lead them into serious trouble after the manic episode is over (e.g., extramarital affairs, quarrels with business associates).
- Patients also might experience an *increase in their cognitive speed*, feeling smarter or more creative than usual.
- Patients with mania usually require *less sleep* than normal, often getting by on only 2 or 3 hours per night.
- Patients might become *more social* and gregarious, going to bars, planning parties, or calling friends at all hours of the night.
- Manic patients tend to talk excessively and manifest *pressured speech*. They answer questions at great length and con-

tinue to talk even when interrupted. Their speech usually is rapid, loud, and emphatic and might manifest as flight of ideas.

- Many manic patients have *psychotic symptoms*, which could include delusions or hallucinations that express themes consistent with the mood, such as delusions about special abilities or powers. Less commonly, the delusions will be mood incongruent and express themes not related to the patient's euphoric and grandiose mood.

Course and outcome. Onset of mania frequently is abrupt, although it might occur gradually over the course of a few weeks. Episodes usually last from a few days to months. They tend to be briefer and have a more abrupt termination than depressive episodes. Risk for recurrence is high. Some patients with bipolar disorder experience good recovery, but a substantial subset of patients continue to have chronic mood instability.

The complications of mania are primarily social: marital discord, divorce, business difficulties, financial extravagance, and sexual indiscretions. Drug or alcohol abuse can occur. If the episode is severe, the patient could be almost completely incapacitated and require hospitalization.

Some patients present with a mixture of manic and depressive symptoms within a single episode of illness. When this occurs, the clinician adds a "with mixed features" specifier to the diagnosis. Typically, a patient with this presentation will have a full manic syndrome that is accompanied by some depressive symptoms, such as feelings of sadness or guilty ruminations. Those with mixed features tend to have an earlier onset, greater number of episodes, higher likelihood of alcohol abuse and suicide attempts, greater likelihood of rapid cycling, and greater likelihood of a lifetime diagnosis of bipolar disorder.

Hypomania

Hypomania is similar to mania but is milder and briefer. During a hypomanic episode, the patient experiences elevated mood and other classic symptoms that define mania, but they are not accompanied by delusional beliefs or hallucinations and are not severe enough to require hospitalization or to impair social and occupational functioning.

Bipolar II disorder is characterized by periods of hypomania that typically occur before or after periods of depression but also might occur independently. These mild manic episodes

TABLE 5–2. DSM-5 depressive and related disorders

Disruptive mood dysregulation disorder

Major depressive disorder, single episode

Major depressive disorder, recurrent

Persistent depressive disorder (dysthymia)

Premenstrual dysphoric disorder

Substance/medication-induced depressive disorder

Depressive disorder due to another medical condition

are not sufficiently severe to require hospitalization, although they can lead to personal, social, or work difficulties. Bipolar II disorder tends to be highly comorbid with other disorders, such as substance use disorders.

Cyclothymic Disorder

Cyclothymic disorder is the mildest form of bipolar disorder and is a condition in which the patient tends to swing from high to low with chronic mild instability of mood.

Depressive Disorders

The DSM-5 depressive disorders are listed in Table 5–2.

Disruptive Mood Dysregulation Disorder

Disruptive mood dysregulation disorder (DMDD) is new to DSM-5 and is characterized by chronic, severe, and persistent irritability in children. The diagnosis recognizes that many children have mood swings, usually from sad to angry, but they do not have bipolar disorder. Many of these children also will have symptoms that meet criteria for oppositional defiant disorder because of overlapping symptoms. In these individuals, the child should be assigned *only* the diagnosis of DMDD.

Children with DMDD stand apart from other boys and girls because of the severity and regularity of their temper outbursts, which tend to be inconsistent with the situation. Between outbursts, the child's mood is persistently irritable or angry, and symptoms are not just a passing phase.

DMDD is common among children presenting to pediatric mental health clinics and occurs mostly in boys. The overall 6-month to 1-year prevalence of DMDD might fall in the range of 2% to 5%. Rates of conversion to bipolar disorder are low. These children are at high risk for depressive and anxiety disorders in adulthood.

Major Depressive Episode

Patients with a major depressive episode must have at least five of nine symptoms of depression, and one of them must be depressed mood or loss of interest or pleasure (see Box 5–2). These characteristic symptoms must be present for at least 2 weeks to rule out transient mood fluctuations. Also, the symptoms must cause clinically significant distress or impairment to differentiate a disorder from normal fluctuations in mood.

Box 5–2. DSM-5 Criteria for Major Depressive Episode

A. Five (or more) of the following symptoms have been present during the same 2-week period and represent a change from previous functioning; at least one of the symptoms is either (1) depressed mood or (2) loss of interest or pleasure.

Note: Do not include symptoms that are clearly attributable to another medical condition.

1. Depressed mood most of the day, nearly every day, as indicated by either subjective report (e.g., feels sad, empty, hopeless) or observation made by others (e.g., appears tearful). (**Note:** In children and adolescents, can be irritable mood.)
2. Markedly diminished interest or pleasure in all, or almost all, activities most of the day, nearly every day (as indicated by either subjective account or observation).
3. Significant weight loss when not dieting or weight gain (e.g., a change of more than 5% of body weight in a month), or decrease or increase in appetite nearly every day. (**Note:** In children, consider failure to make expected weight gain.)
4. Insomnia or hypersomnia nearly every day.
5. Psychomotor agitation or retardation nearly every day (observable by others, not merely subjective feelings of restlessness or being slowed down).
6. Fatigue or loss of energy nearly every day.
7. Feelings of worthlessness or excessive or inappropriate guilt (which may be delusional) nearly every day (not merely self-reproach or guilt about being sick).

8. Diminished ability to think or concentrate, or indecisiveness, nearly every day (either by subjective account or as observed by others).
9. Recurrent thoughts of death (not just fear of dying), recurrent suicidal ideation without a specific plan, or a suicide attempt or a specific plan for committing suicide.

B. The symptoms cause clinically significant distress or impairment in social, occupational, or other important areas of functioning.

C. The episode is not attributable to the physiological effects of a substance or another medical condition.

Note: Criteria A–C represent a major depressive episode.

Note: Responses to a significant loss (e.g., bereavement, financial ruin, losses from a natural disaster, a serious medical illness or disability) may include the feelings of intense sadness, rumination about the loss, insomnia, poor appetite, and weight loss noted in Criterion A, which may resemble a depressive episode. Although such symptoms may be understandable or considered appropriate to the loss, the presence of a major depressive episode in addition to the normal response to a significant loss should also be carefully considered. This decision inevitably requires the exercise of clinical judgment based on the individual's history and the cultural norms for the expression of distress in the context of loss.[1]

---

[1]In distinguishing grief from a major depressive episode (MDE), it is useful to consider that in grief the predominant affect is feelings of emptiness and loss, while in an MDE it is persistent depressed mood and the inability to anticipate happiness or pleasure. The dysphoria in grief is likely to decrease in intensity over days to weeks and occurs in waves, the so-called pangs of grief. These waves tend to be associated with thoughts or reminders of the deceased. The depressed mood of an MDE is more persistent and not tied to specific thoughts or preoccupations. The pain of grief may be accompanied by positive emotions and humor that are uncharacteristic of the pervasive unhappiness and misery characteristic of an MDE. The thought content associated with grief generally features a preoccupation with thoughts and memories of the deceased, rather than the self-critical or pessimistic ruminations seen in an MDE. In grief, self-esteem is generally preserved, whereas in an MDE feelings of worthlessness and self-loathing are common. If self-derogatory ideation is present in grief, it typically involves perceived failings vis-à-vis the deceased (e.g., not visiting frequently enough, not telling the deceased how much he or she was loved). If a bereaved individual thinks about death and dying, such thoughts are generally focused on the deceased and possibly about "joining" the deceased, whereas in an MDE such thoughts are focused on ending one's own life because of feeling worthless, undeserving of life, or unable to cope with the pain of depression.

Because major depressive disorder is the most common psychiatric illness that clinicians are likely to encounter, it is worthwhile to commit the nine characteristic symptoms to memory. When interviewing patients to determine whether they are depressed, the clinician must mentally run through this list of symptoms. This can be facilitated through the use of the simple mnemonic, **SIGECAPS: S**leep decreased, **I**nterest decreased, **G**uilt or worthlessness, **E**nergy decreased, **C**oncentration difficulties, **A**ppetite disturbance, **P**sychomotor retardation, **S**uicidal thoughts.

Clinical findings.   The person who is depressed feels sad, despondent, down in the dumps, or full of despair. Some patients will report feeling tense or irritable, with only a small component of sadness, or of having lost their ability to feel pleasure or experience interest in things they normally enjoy.

The depressive syndrome may be accompanied by a group of *vegetative* symptoms, such as decreased appetite or insomnia. Decreased appetite often leads to some weight loss, although some depressed persons will force themselves to eat despite decreased appetite, or might be urged to eat by a parent or spouse. Less frequently, depression expresses itself as a desire to eat excessively and is accompanied by weight gain. Insomnia is common and could be initial, middle, or terminal. *Initial insomnia* means that the patient has difficulty falling asleep, often tossing or turning for several hours before dozing off. *Middle insomnia* refers to awakening in the middle of the night, remaining awake for an hour or two, and finally falling asleep again. *Terminal insomnia* refers to awakening early in the morning and being unable to return to sleep.

Other symptoms of depression include the following:

- *Motor activity alteration.* Patients with psychomotor retardation might sit quietly in a chair for hours without speaking to anyone, simply staring into space. Conversely, patients with psychomotor agitation are restless and seem extremely nervous. They are unable to sit in a chair and frequently pace about the room.
- *Fatiguing too easily or lacking energy.* In a primary care setting, this may be one of the most common presenting complaints of depression.
- *Feelings of worthlessness and guilt.* Depressed persons may lose confidence in themselves so that they are fearful of going to work, taking examinations, or assuming responsibility for household tasks.

- *Difficulty concentrating or thinking.* Patients with depression feel that they function less effectively at work, are unable to study, or in severe cases are even unable to perform simple cognitive tasks such as watching a show on television or reading.
- *Thoughts of death or dying.* Suicide may be seen either as an escape from their suffering or as a deserved punishment for their various misdeeds.
- *Diurnal variation in mood.* Typically, patients state that their mood is worse in the morning but improves as the day progresses, so that they feel best in the evening. Sometimes patients report the reverse pattern.
- *Delusions or hallucinations.* These usually are congruent with the depressed mood ("mood-congruent"). Less often, the delusions will be inconsistent with depressed mood ("mood-incongruent").

Course and outcome. A depressive episode might begin either suddenly or gradually. The duration of an untreated episode could range from a few weeks to months or even years, although most depressive episodes clear spontaneously within approximately 6 months. The prognosis for any single depressive episode is quite good, particularly in view of the efficacy of the available treatment. Unfortunately, most patients will have a recurrence of depression at some time in their lives, with approximately 20% developing a chronic form of depression.

Suicide is the most serious outcome. An estimated 10%–15% of severely ill depressed patients will take their own lives. Persons at heightened risk include those who are divorced or live alone, have a history of substance abuse, are over age 40, have a history of a prior suicide attempt(s), or express suicidal ideation. Suicide and suicidal behavior are discussed in detail in Chapter 18.

Persistent Depressive Disorder

Persistent depressive disorder, formerly *dysthymic disorder*, is a chronic and persistent disturbance in mood that has been present for at least 2 years (at least one year for children and adolescents) and is characterized by relatively typical depressive symptoms such as anorexia, insomnia, decreased energy, low self-esteem, difficulty concentrating, and feelings of hopelessness. Because this is a chronic, mild disorder, only two of six symptoms are necessary, but they must have persisted more or less continuously for at least a 2-year period. Major depressive disorder might precede persistent depressive disorder, and major depressive episodes could occur during persistent depressive disorder. Individuals whose symptoms meet major depressive disorder criteria for 2 years should receive a diagnosis of persistent depressive disorder in addition to major depressive disorder.

Persistent depressive disorder often has an early onset, typically in childhood, adolescence, or early adult life, and by definition is chronic. Early onset (i.e., before age 21) is associated with a higher likelihood of comorbid personality disorders and substance use disorders.

Patients with persistent depressive disorder are chronically unhappy and miserable. Some also develop the relatively more severe major depressive syndrome. When the major depressive episode clears, these patients usually return to their chronic low mood.

Premenstrual Dysphoric Disorder

Premenstrual dysphoric disorder is a new diagnosis in DSM-5. The disorder is common and causes significant distress and impairment. Clinical research and epidemiological studies have shown that many women experience depressive symptoms that begin during the luteal phase of the menstrual cycle and terminate around the onset of menses. Additionally, these studies identify a subset of women (approximately 2%) who suffer intermittently from severe symptoms associated with the luteal phase of the menstrual cycle.

Mood Disorder Specifiers

The mood disorders can be further subdivided based on patterns of symptoms detected during a careful evaluation. DSM-5 recognizes the following specifiers:

- *Anxious distress* is a prominent feature of both bipolar disorder and major depressive disorder. High levels of anxiety are associated with higher suicide risk, longer duration of illness, and greater likelihood of treatment nonresponse.
- *Mixed features* that occur with a major depressive episode have been found to be a significant risk factor for developing bipolar I or bipolar II disorder.
- *Melancholic features* describes a relatively severe form of depression that may be more likely to respond to medication or electroconvulsive therapy (ECT). Melancholia requires

the presence of one of two specific features: loss of pleasure and inability to respond to pleasurable stimuli. At least three from a list of six additional features also are required: distinct quality of depressed mood, depression that is regularly worse in the morning (diurnal variation), early morning awakening (terminal insomnia), marked psychomotor agitation or retardation, significant anorexia or weight loss, and excessive or inappropriate guilt.

- *Atypical features* manifest as weight gain and hypersomnia. In addition, patients with these features are quite responsive to their life situation. The individual's *mood reactivity* is the capacity to be easily cheered by positive events (e.g., an unexpected compliment, a visit from one's children) but to feel devastated by perceived slights or rejections. Monoamine oxidase inhibitors (MAOIs) have proved particularly useful with this group of patients.
- *Psychotic features* identify those patients with delusions or hallucinations. The content of the delusions or hallucinations is either consistent or not consistent with typical depressive themes, or a combination.
- *Catatonia* identifies a subgroup of patients who have catatonic features similar to those that have been observed in schizophrenia (e.g., posturing, waxy flexibility, catalepsy, negativism, and mutism).
- *Peripartum onset* identifies patients who experience a depressive, manic, or hypomanic episode during pregnancy or within the first 4 weeks postpartum.
- *Seasonal pattern* identifies persons with depression typically occurring more frequently during the winter months and in whom remission of the depression or switches from depression to mania occur during a characteristic time of year (e.g., in the spring). Light therapy can be an effective treatment for seasonal affective disorder (i.e., depressive illness that recurs in winter months and tends to remit in the spring). The U.S. Food and Drug Administration (FDA) has approved an extended-release form of bupropion as a treatment for those with seasonal affective disorder.
- *Rapid cycling* identifies those patients who have had at least four mood episodes (i.e., major depressive, manic, hypomanic), occurring in any combination or order, during the past 12 months. Rapid-cycling bipolar disorder is associated with a younger age at onset, more frequent depressive episodes, and greater risk for suicide attempts than other forms of the disorder.

Differential Diagnosis

The clinician should always rule out drugs of abuse, sedatives, tranquilizers, antihypertensives, oral contraceptives, and glucocorticoids as causes of mania or depression. General medical conditions such as hypothyroidism and systemic lupus erythematosus also can manifest with prominent depressive symptoms. In these cases, treatment usually involves withdrawing or reducing the drug or treating the underlying medical illness.

Dysphoric mood also can occur in schizophrenia. In schizophrenia the dysphoric mood typically is apathetic or empty, whereas in depression the dysphoric mood usually is experienced as intensely painful. Patients with schizophrenia and those with major depressive disorder both could experience psychotic symptoms; therefore, severe psychotic depression sometimes is difficult to distinguish from schizophrenia. When psychotic symptoms persist after mood symptoms remit, a diagnosis of schizophrenia or schizoaffective disorder is more likely.

The differential diagnosis between mania and schizophrenia also is quite important. Several features are useful in making this distinction. Personality and general functioning usually are satisfactory before and after a manic episode, even though mild disturbances in mood can occur. Although manic episodes could manifest with disorganized speech, speech abnormalities in mania are always accompanied by a disturbance in mood and usually by overactivity and physical agitation. Patients with mania could experience delusions or hallucinations, but these typically are mood-congruent. Additional features that make the diagnosis of manic episode more likely include a family history of a mood disorder, good premorbid adjustment, and a previous episode of a mood disorder from which the patient completely or substantially recovered. When psychotic symptoms persist in the absence of an abnormality in mood, a diagnosis of schizophrenia or schizoaffective disorder is more likely.

People facing *bereavement* might present with many depressive symptoms and the symptoms might have been present long enough to meet the criteria for a major depressive episode. In DSM-5, these individuals are now diagnosed with major depressive disorder.

Epidemiology

The National Comorbidity Study reported a lifetime prevalence of nearly 17% for major depressive disorder and about 2% for bipolar I and II disorders combined. Persistent depressive disorder has a prevalence of approximately 2%–3%. Combined, these disorders affect more than one in five persons. Depression is more common in women than in men, with a ratio of approximately 2:1 in the United States. Bipolar disorder also is more common in women than in men, with a ratio of approximately 3:2. The median age at onset for major depressive disorder is 32 years; for bipolar disorder, 25 years; and for dysthymia, 31 years. Men tend to have an earlier onset of bipolar disorder compared with women.

Treatment

Mania

Lithium, valproate, and carbamazepine are all FDA-approved for treating acute mania. Lamotrigine is approved for maintenance treatment of bipolar disorder. Several other anticonvulsant drugs (including gabapentin and topiramate) have been used to treat patients with bipolar disorder, but studies have produced mixed results. In addition, nearly all second-generation antipsychotics are approved to treat acute mania (except clozapine), and several have received indications for maintenance treatment of bipolar disorder or as adjuncts to lithium or valproate. ECT is highly effective for treating mania when medication is ineffective.

Clinical Points for Mania

- Use somatic therapies aggressively to treat manic symptoms as rapidly as possible.

- Follow the patient closely as the mania "breaks" to determine whether a subsequent depression is emerging.

- After an episode of mania, patients should receive maintenance medication; typically, they will continue to take mood stabilizers for several years, and perhaps for the remainder of their lives, to prevent relapses.

- Advise patients about the importance of getting sufficient sleep and following sensible sleep hygiene measures (described in Chapter 12).

- Even when patients are stable, follow up with them regularly to ensure continued compliance with medication and to monitor blood levels (if applicable).

- Manic episodes can have devastating personal, social, and economic consequences; patients will usually require (at a minimum) supportive psychotherapy to help them cope with these consequences and maintain their self-esteem.

- Provide family members with both psychological support, as needed, and educational materials to help them understand the disorder, its symptoms, and the need for continued treatment.

- Patients with bipolar illness often are appreciative of being told about the "good side" of their illness: its association with creativity and high achievement.

Depression

Pharmacotherapy

Several medications are available to treat depression: tricyclics and other related compounds, MAOIs, selective serotonin reuptake inhibitors (SSRIs), and other antidepressants that are not easily categorized (e.g., bupropion, mirtazapine, vilazodone). These drugs are all thought to work by altering levels of various neurotransmitters at crucial nerve terminals in the central nervous system. Antidepressants are largely similar in their overall effectiveness, and from 65%–70% of persons who receive antidepressants will improve markedly. Unfortunately, and despite adequate treatment, some patients never fully respond or have only minimal improvement.

Begin treatment with an SSRI, because agents in this medication class are well tolerated and safe in overdose. Low dosages generally are effective, and frequent dosage adjustments usually are unnecessary. Patients with cardiac conduction defects should receive an SSRI, bupropion, or another one of the newer medications (e.g., vilazodone, vortioxetine). Impulsive or suicidal patients should receive an SSRI or one of the newer medications that are unlikely to be dangerous in overdose. Most patients will improve relatively quickly, even within the first 1–2 weeks after starting medication. Because antidepressants have been reported to increase the risk for impulsive behavior and suicidal behaviors in teenagers and young adults, carefully monitor patients.

Drug trials generally should last 4–8 weeks. If the patient fails to respond within 4 weeks, increase the dosage or switch the patient to another medication, preferably from another drug class (e.g., providing a different balance of norepinephrine, serotonin, and acetylcholine).

If response is not optimal, adding lithium ("augmentation") is the best-researched option to boost the effectiveness of an antidepressant. Other agents used for augmentation include triiodothyronine, a thyroid preparation; psychostimulants such as methylphenidate; pindolol, a beta-blocker; and benzodiazepines. The antipsychotic aripiprazole is FDA-approved for this purpose.

When a depressed patient is psychotic, the best strategy is to co-administer an antipsychotic with an antidepressant. Benzodiazepines co-administered with the antidepressant could help calm an anxious or agitated patient with depression relatively quickly.

For patients who are experiencing their first episode of depression, continue the drug for another 16–36 weeks after the patient is considered to have recovered. Thereafter, the clinician could decide to discontinue the medication while monitoring the patient closely.

Discontinue the medication gradually, because many patients experience mild withdrawal symptoms, particularly if tricyclics or SSRIs (except fluoxetine) are discontinued abruptly. Symptoms that can occur during antidepressant withdrawal include insomnia and nervousness, nightmares, and gastrointestinal symptoms such as nausea or vomiting. Patients with recurrent depression often will need long-term maintenance, typically at the full treatment dosage. Long-term maintenance treatment can significantly reduce the risk of relapse and improve the patient's quality of life.

MAOIs can be used to treat patients whose symptoms do not respond to first-line antidepressants or those unable to tolerate their adverse effects. MAOIs should be used with caution because they potentially have more dangerous adverse effects and interactions than do other antidepressants.

Mood Disorders   **91**

ECT is another treatment option for depression. ECT often produces a rapid remission of depressive symptoms. Patients will need maintenance antidepressant treatment after a course of ECT. Repetitive transcranial magnetic stimulation and vagal nerve stimulation are newer treatments for depression, but neither is widely available.

Psychotherapy

Some depressed patients will respond well to brief psychotherapy alone. Cognitive-behavioral therapy and interpersonal psychotherapy are as effective as medication for treating mild to moderately severe depression, and their combination with psychotherapy is even more powerful. These are described more fully in Chapter 20.

Clinical Points for Depression

- Establish a hopeful, optimistic tone at the initial interview.

  - Assess the severity of the depressive syndrome, remembering that there might be individual and cultural differences in the way depression is experienced and expressed.

  - Do not attempt extensive psychological probing when the patient is deeply depressed.

  - Determine suicide risk initially and reassess frequently.

- Aggressively treat moderate to severe depression with somatic therapy.

  - Severely depressed or suicidal patients might require hospitalization.

  - Severely depressed outpatients might need frequent (e.g., twice-weekly) brief (e.g., 10- to 15-minute) contacts for support and medication management until their depression lifts.

  - Most patients will require at least 16–36 weeks of maintenance medication after an initial episode and thereafter should be given a trial of decreasing or discontinuing the medication. If symptoms reemerge, reinstitute the medication and consider long-term drug administration.

- Determine whether psychosocial stressors are present that are contributing to the depressed mood and counsel the patient on ways to cope with them.

- Depressed patients tend to "get down" on themselves because they have been depressed; help the patient to learn to abandon negative or self-deprecating attitudes through cognitive-behavioral therapy or other psychotherapeutic techniques.

Further Reading

American Psychiatric Association: Practice guideline for the treatment of patients with bipolar disorder (revision). Am J Psychiatry 159(4, suppl):1–50, 2002

American Psychiatric Association: Practice Guideline for the Treatment of Patients With Major Depressive Disorder, 3rd Edition. Arlington, VA, American Psychiatric Association, 2010

Goldberg JF, Perlis RH, Bowden CL, et al: Manic symptoms during depressive episodes in 1,380 patients with bipolar disorder: findings from the STEP-BD. Am J Psychiatry 166(2):173–181, 2009

Goodwin FK, Jamison KR: Manic-Depressive Illness: Bipolar Disorders and Recurrent Depression, 2nd Edition. New York, Oxford University Press, 2007

Hollon SD, DeRubeis RJ, Fawcett J, et al: Effect of cognitive therapy with antidepressant medications vs antidepressants alone on the rate of recovery in major depressive disorder: a randomized clinical trial. JAMA Psychiatry 71(10):1157–1164, 2014

Kennedy SH, Giacobbe P: Treatment resistant depression—advances in somatic therapies. Ann Clin Psychiatry 19(4):279–287, 2007

Ketter TA (ed): Handbook of Diagnosis and Treatment of Bipolar Disorder. Washington, DC, American Psychiatric Publishing, 2010

Klein DN, Schwartz JE, Rose S, Leader JB: Five-year course and outcome of dysthymic disorder: A prospective, naturalistic follow-up study. Am J Psychiatry 157(6):931–939, 2000

Li X, Frye MA, Shelton RC: Review of pharmacological treatment in mood disorders and future directions for drug development. Neuropsychopharmacology 37(1):77–101, 2012

Nemeroff CB: The role of corticotropin-releasing factor in the pathogenesis of major depression. Pharmacopsychiatry 21(2):76–82, 1988

Pampallona S, Bollini P, Tibaldi G, et al: Combined pharmacotherapy and psychological treatment for depression: a systematic review. Arch Gen Psychiatry 61(7):714–719, 2004

Quitkin FM, McGrath PJ, Stewart JW, et al: Remission rates with 3 consecutive antidepressant trials: effectiveness for depressed outpatients. J Clin Psychiatry 66(6):670–676, 2005

Rosa MA, Lisanby SH: Somatic treatments for mood disorders. Neuropsychopharmacology 37(1):102–116, 2012

Schneck CD, Miklowitz DJ, Miyahara S, et al: The prospective course of rapid-cycling bipolar disorder: findings from the STEP-BD. Am J Psychiatry 165(3):370–377, quiz 410, 2008

Trivedi MH, Thase ME, Fava M, et al: Adjunctive aripiprazole in major depressive disorder: analysis of efficacy and safety in patients with anxious and atypical features. J Clin Psychiatry 69(12):1928–1936, 2008

Chapter 6

Anxiety Disorders

Anxiety disorders are among the most common psychiatric conditions worldwide and are a leading cause of distress and impairment. The word *anxiety* refers to the presence of fear or apprehension that is out of proportion to the situation. Anxiety disorders have been reconceptualized in DSM-5, and posttraumatic stress disorder and obsessive-compulsive disorder have been split off into their own chapters, while separation anxiety disorder and selective mutism are new to the chapter. The DSM-5 anxiety disorders are listed in Table 6–1.

Separation Anxiety Disorder

With separation anxiety disorder, a person has excessive anxiety regarding separation from places or people to whom he or she has a strong emotional attachment. The 12-month estimated prevalence of separation anxiety disorder is approximately 4% in children and 1%–2% in adults. Most adults with separation anxiety disorder experienced first onset during adulthood. In children, the strong emotional attachment likely is to a parent, but in adults the attachment might be to a spouse or friend. The DSM-5 criteria for separation anxiety disorder are shown in Box 6–1.

Box 6–1.   DSM-5 Criteria for Separation Anxiety Disorder

A. Developmentally inappropriate and excessive fear or anxiety concerning separation from those to whom the individual is attached, as evidenced by at least three of the following:

1. Recurrent excessive distress when anticipating or experiencing separation from home or from major attachment figures.

2. Persistent and excessive worry about losing major attachment figures or about possible harm to them, such as illness, injury, disasters, or death.
3. Persistent and excessive worry about experiencing an untoward event (e.g., getting lost, being kidnapped, having an accident, becoming ill) that causes separation from a major attachment figure.
4. Persistent reluctance or refusal to go out, away from home, to school, to work, or elsewhere because of fear of separation.
5. Persistent and excessive fear of or reluctance about being alone or without major attachment figures at home or in other settings.
6. Persistent reluctance or refusal to sleep away from home or to go to sleep without being near a major attachment figure.
7. Repeated nightmares involving the theme of separation.
8. Repeated complaints of physical symptoms (e.g., headaches, stomachaches, nausea, vomiting) when separation from major attachment figures occurs or is anticipated.

B. The fear, anxiety, or avoidance is persistent, lasting at least 4 weeks in children and adolescents and typically 6 months or more in adults.

C. The disturbance causes clinically significant distress or impairment in social, academic, occupational, or other important areas of functioning.

D. The disturbance is not better explained by another mental disorder, such as refusing to leave home because of excessive resistance to change in autism spectrum disorder; delusions or hallucinations concerning separation in psychotic disorders; refusal to go outside without a trusted companion in agoraphobia; worries about ill health or other harm befalling significant others in generalized anxiety disorder; or concerns about having an illness in illness anxiety disorder.

In children, this disorder could present as *school phobia*, school refusal, or school absenteeism. Some children develop a fear of going to school, typically during grade school or junior high school. A child who previously has been attending school begins to develop excuses for staying home, such as repeated episodes of "illness" involving, for example, headache or nausea, while others may be truant. Not all children who refuse to attend school have separation anxiety disorder, and for that reason clinicians need to rule out other diagnostic possibilities (e.g., truancy secondary to conduct disorder,

TABLE 6–1. DSM-5 anxiety disorders

Separation anxiety disorder

Selective mutism

Specific phobia

Social anxiety disorder (social phobia)

Panic disorder

Agoraphobia

Generalized anxiety disorder

Substance/medication-induced anxiety disorder

Anxiety disorder due to another medical condition

---

avoidance of school as a complication of mood disorder or secondary to psychosis) or even stressors such as bullying.

Treating separation anxiety disorder involves a combination of medication and individual psychotherapy, often with family therapy or parental guidance. Selective serotonin reuptake inhibitors (SSRIs) have been used to help control feelings of anxiety and fear, as have benzodiazepines. Cognitive-behavioral therapy (CBT) can help the child or adult to correct dysfunctional beliefs (e.g., "No one likes me"), promote a positive self-image, and learn problem-solving skills. This can be combined with social skills training, graded exposure and desensitization, and anxiety reduction techniques (e.g., relaxation training). Parental involvement can help reinforce the child's successes, promote the child's social participation, and model appropriate behavior.

Selective Mutism

Selective mutism is the persistent failure to speak in specific social situations where speaking is expected despite being able to speak in other situations (e.g., at home). The disorder is uncommon and most likely to manifest in young children. Selective mutism can cause significant impairment. As these children mature, they might face increasing social isolation and in school settings suffer academic impairment, because often they do not communicate appropriately with teachers regarding academic or personal needs. Brief periods of selective silence lasting less than a month do not qualify an individual for this diagnosis.

Selective mutism should be distinguished from speech disturbances that are better explained by a communication disorder, such as language disorder, speech sound disorder (previously phonological disorder), childhood-onset fluency disorder (stuttering), or pragmatic (social) communication disorder.

Treatment of selective mutism is difficult and usually involves use of SSRIs and CBT. Parents and teachers often make accommodations for the child's muteness, but it generally is useful to maintain the expectation that the child will talk and communicate, at least for a certain amount of time at home and at school.

Specific Phobia and Social Anxiety Disorder

Phobias are irrational fears of specific objects, places or situations, or activities. With *social anxiety disorder* (formerly *social phobia*), the individual tends to fear performance situations such as speaking in public, eating in restaurants, writing in front of other persons, or using public restrooms. Sometimes the fear becomes generalized, so that phobic persons avoid most social situations. *Specific phobias* usually are well circumscribed and involve fearing objects that could cause harm, such as snakes, heights, flying, or blood.

For these diagnoses, DSM-5 requires that the phobia must have lasted at least 6 months, a requirement meant to exclude individuals with transient fears. The phobia must cause clinically significant distress or impairment, and other causes for the disorder, including another mental disorder or medical condition, must be ruled out. Patients with social phobia are ill at ease in the interview situation and often appear anxious or fearful. Their verbal responses might be restricted. With specific phobia, the clinician can specify type: animal, natural environment (e.g., storms), blood-injection-injury, situational (e.g., airplanes), or other. For social anxiety disorder, the clinician can specify if the disorder is "performance only" if it is restricted to speaking or performing in public.

Epidemiology and Clinical Findings

Specific phobias and social anxiety disorder are surprisingly common, with prevalence rates in the National Comorbidity Survey of 11% for specific phobias and 13% for social anxiety disorder. Specific phobias are more common in women, whereas social anxiety disorder affects men and women equally. Specific phobias begin in childhood, with most starting before age 12. Social anxiety disorder emerges during adolescence, and almost always before age 25. The most common specific phobias involve animals, storms, heights, illness, injury, and death.

Social anxiety disorder tends to develop slowly, is chronic, and has no obvious precipitating events. Whether the disorder is perceived as disabling depends on the nature and extent of the fear as well as one's occupation and social position. A business executive whose job requires meeting with the public, for example, would face greater disability from social anxiety disorder than would a software designer who works in isolation. About one in eight persons with social anxiety disorder develops a substance use disorder, and approximately one-half have symptoms that meet criteria for another psychiatric disorder, such as major depression.

Etiology and Pathophysiology

Phobic disorders tend to run in families. Studies show that relatives of phobic persons are significantly more likely to have phobias than those of controls. The disorders tend to "breed true"—that is, people with social anxiety disorder are likely to have relatives with social anxiety disorder, not a specific phobia.

The biological underpinnings of the phobias are not well understood. Research suggests that dopaminergic pathways play a role in social anxiety disorder. Patients with this disorder show a preferential response to monoamine oxidase inhibitors (MAOIs), which have dopaminergic activity. Lower levels of dopamine metabolites in cerebrospinal fluid have been linked to introversion, a facet of social anxiety disorder. In addition, functional brain imaging studies have found decreased striatal dopamine D_2 receptor and dopamine transporter binding in patients with social anxiety disorder.

Learning also might play an important role in the etiology of phobias. Behaviorists have noted that many phobias arise in association with traumatic events (e.g., developing a fear of heights after a fall).

Differential Diagnosis

The differential diagnosis of phobic disorders includes other anxiety disorders (e.g., panic disorder), obsessive-compulsive disorder, mood disorders, and avoidant personality disorder. A person with obsessive-compulsive disorder typically has multiple fears and phobias, not isolated, circumscribed fears. The distinction between avoidant personality disorder and social anxiety disorder is difficult. Generally, a person with avoidant personality disorder does not fear specific social situations but feels insecure about social relationships and fears being hurt by others.

Clinical Management

Fluoxetine (10–30 mg/day), paroxetine (20–50 mg/day), sertraline (50–200 mg/day), and a long-acting formulation of venlafaxine (75–225 mg/day) are all FDA-approved for treating social anxiety disorder. Other SSRIs probably are also effective, as are the MAOIs and benzodiazepines, but not tricyclic antidepressants (TCAs). Patients tend to relapse when the drugs are discontinued. Beta-blocking drugs are effective for short-term treatment of performance-related anxiety but otherwise are ineffective. Medication generally is ineffective for treating specific phobias, although benzodiazepines can provide short-term benefit.

CBT can be effective in the treatment of social anxiety disorder and specific phobias. The patient is exposed to the feared situation or object through the techniques of systematic desensitization and flooding. In the former, patients are gradually exposed to feared situations, beginning with the one they fear the least. With flooding, patients are instructed to enter situations that are associated with anxiety until the anxiety associated with the exposure (e.g., eating in restaurants) subsides.

Panic Disorder

Panic disorder consists of recurrent, unexpected panic (or anxiety) attacks that are distressing, upsetting, and cause persistent worry or change one's behavior. The DSM-5 diagnostic criteria for panic disorder are shown in Box 6–2.

Box 6–2.   DSM-5 Criteria for Panic Disorder

A. Recurrent unexpected panic attacks. A panic attack is an abrupt surge of intense fear or intense discomfort that reaches a peak within minutes, and during which time four (or more) of the following symptoms occur:

Note: The abrupt surge can occur from a calm state or an anxious state.

1. Palpitations, pounding heart, or accelerated heart rate.
2. Sweating.
3. Trembling or shaking.
4. Sensations of shortness of breath or smothering.
5. Feelings of choking.
6. Chest pain or discomfort.
7. Nausea or abdominal distress.
8. Feeling dizzy, unsteady, light-headed, or faint.
9. Chills or heat sensations.
10. Paresthesias (numbness or tingling sensations).
11. Derealization (feelings of unreality) or depersonalization (being detached from oneself).
12. Fear of losing control or "going crazy."
13. Fear of dying.

Note: Culture-specific symptoms (e.g., tinnitus, neck soreness, headache, uncontrollable screaming or crying) may be seen. Such symptoms should not count as one of the four required symptoms.

B. At least one of the attacks has been followed by 1 month (or more) of one or both of the following:

1. Persistent concern or worry about additional panic attacks or their consequences (e.g., losing control, having a heart attack, "going crazy").
2. A significant maladaptive change in behavior related to the attacks (e.g., behaviors designed to avoid having panic attacks, such as avoidance of exercise or unfamiliar situations).

C. The disturbance is not attributable to the physiological effects of a substance (e.g., a drug of abuse, a medication) or another medical condition (e.g., hyperthyroidism, cardiopulmonary disorders).

D. The disturbance is not better explained by another mental disorder (e.g., the panic attacks do not occur only in response to feared social situations, as in social anxiety disorder; in response to circumscribed phobic objects or situations, as in specific phobia; in response to obsessions, as in obsessive-compulsive disorder; in response to reminders of traumatic events, as in posttraumatic stress disorder; or in response to separation from attachment figures, as in separation anxiety disorder).

Epidemiology and Clinical Findings

Approximately 5% of women and 2% of men have symptoms that meet criteria for panic disorder at some point in their lives. Panic disorder has onset during a patient's mid-20s, and nearly 8 in 10 develop the disorder before age 30. Often there are no precipitating stressors before onset. The initial panic attack usually is alarming and could prompt a visit to an emergency department. Many patients undergo extensive and medically unnecessary workups that focus on the target symptoms.

Panic attacks develop suddenly, typically peaking within 10 minutes. During attacks, patients hyperventilate and appear fearful, pale, diaphoretic, and restless. Many patients report that their attacks last hours to days, but it is likely that their continuing symptoms represent anxiety that persists after an attack. Common symptoms are presented in Table 6–2.

Panic disorder usually is chronic but fluctuates in frequency and severity. Most patients with panic disorder improve, but complete remission is not common. Panic disorder patients are at increased risk for peptic ulcer disease and cardiovascular disease, including hypertension, and have higher death rates than the general population, including from suicide. The most common comorbid psychiatric disorders are major depression and alcohol use disorder.

Etiology and Pathophysiology

Family and twin studies strongly suggest that panic disorder is hereditary. The morbidity risk for panic disorder is nearly 20% among first-degree relatives compared with only 2% among control relatives. Twin studies show higher concordance rates for panic disorder among identical twins than among nonidentical twins, which is evidence that genetic influences predominate over environmental influences. Molecular genetic studies targeting genes thought to be associated with fear and anxiety are under way.

Among the biological mechanisms possibly underlying panic disorder are increased catecholamine levels in the cen-

TABLE 6–2. Common symptoms of panic disorder

Symptoms	%	Symptoms	%
Fearfulness or worry	96	Restlessness	80
Nervousness	95	Trouble breathing	80
Palpitations	93	Easy fatigability	76
Muscle aching or tension	89	Trouble concentrating	76
Trembling or shaking	89	Irritability	74
Apprehension	83	Trouble sleeping	74
Dizziness or imbalance	82	Chest pain or discomfort	69
Fear of dying or going crazy	81	Numbness or tingling	65
Faintness/light-headedness	80	Tendency to startle	57
Hot or cold sensations	80	Choking or smothering sensations	54

tral nervous system, an abnormality in the locus coeruleus (an area of the brain stem regulating alertness), carbon dioxide hypersensitivity, a disturbance in lactate metabolism, and abnormalities of the γ-aminobutyric acid (GABA) neurotransmitter system.

Differential Diagnosis

The symptoms of panic attacks sometimes are caused by medical conditions, including hyperthyroidism, pheochromocytoma, diseases of the vestibular nerve, hypoglycemia, and supraventricular tachycardia. These diagnostic possibilities must be ruled out (Table 6–3).

Patients with major depressive disorder often develop anxiety and panic attacks, which resolve when the depression is treated. Panic attacks also could occur in patients with generalized anxiety disorder (GAD), schizophrenia, depersonalization disorder, somatization disorder, and borderline personality disorder.

In DSM-5, the presence of isolated panic attacks can be specified by indicating their presence ("with panic attacks") in patients with other conditions.

TABLE 6–3. Differential diagnosis of panic disorder and other anxiety disorders

Medical illnesses	Drugs
Angina	Caffeine
Cardiac arrhythmias	Aminophylline and related compounds
Congestive heart failure	
Hypoglycemia	Sympathomimetic agents (e.g., decongestants and diet pills)
Hypoxia	Monosodium glutamate
Pulmonary embolism	Psychostimulants and hallucinogens withdrawal
Severe pain	
Thyrotoxicosis	Withdrawal from benzodiazepines and other sedative-hypnotics
Carcinoid	
Pheochromocytoma	
Menière's disease	Thyroid hormones
	Antipsychotic medication
Psychiatric illnesses	
Schizophrenia	
Mood disorders	
Avoidant personality disorder	
Adjustment disorder with anxious mood	

Clinical Management

SSRIs effectively block panic attacks in 70%–80% of patients. The FDA has approved fluoxetine, paroxetine, and sertraline for treating panic disorder. A long-acting formulation of the serotonin-norepinephrine reuptake inhibitor (SNRI) venlafaxine also is FDA-approved. Antidepressant dosage depends on the specific medication but usually is similar to dosages used to treat major depression. After panic attacks have remitted, the patient should continue taking medication for at least 1 year to prevent relapse.

TCAs and MAOIs are effective but are rarely used. Beta-blocking drugs, such as propranolol, sometimes are prescribed but are much less effective than SSRIs. Benzodiazepines can be effective in blocking panic attacks, but they could be habit-forming.

Patients should avoid caffeine because it can induce anxiety. Patients often do not realize how much caffeine they are ingesting with coffee (50–150 mg), tea (20–50 mg), cola drinks (30–60 mg), and even milk chocolate (1–15 mg).

CBT is effective for treating panic disorder and often is combined with medication. CBT usually involves distraction and breathing exercises, along with educating patients about how to appropriately attribute distressing somatic symptoms.

Agoraphobia

Agoraphobia is characterized by avoidance of places or situations from which a quick escape is difficult in the event of a panic attack. As a consequence of this fear, the individual with agoraphobia avoids places or situations where this might occur ("phobic avoidance"). DSM-5 criteria require that the person have marked fear or anxiety of two or more situations (e.g., using public transportation, being in open spaces); that he or she avoid these places because escape might be difficult; and that the agoraphobic situation almost always provoke fear. The fear, anxiety, or avoidance of the situation is persistent, typically lasting more than 6 months, and is not due to another medical condition or mental disorder.

Agoraphobia often occurs as a complication of panic disorder. Agoraphobia is nearly as common as panic disorder; women are more likely than men to develop agoraphobia. When panic disorder and agoraphobia are both present, each disorder should be diagnosed.

The term *agoraphobia* translates literally from Greek as "fear of the marketplace." Although many agoraphobia patients are uncomfortable in shops and markets, their true fear is being separated from a source of security. Agoraphobia patients tend to avoid crowded places, such as malls, restaurants, theaters, and churches, because they feel trapped. Many agoraphobia patients are able to go places they might otherwise avoid if accompanied by a trusted person or even a pet. Some individuals with severe agoraphobia are unable to leave their home.

Common situations that either provoke or relieve anxiety in people with agoraphobia are shown in Table 6–4.

Because many people with agoraphobia will have panic disorder, medication usually is recommended, with the agents

TABLE 6–4. Common situations that either provoke or relieve anxiety (percentage of sample of 100 agoraphobia patients)

Situations that provoke anxiety	%	Situations that relieve anxiety	%
Standing in line at a store	96	Being accompanied by spouse	85
Having an appointment	91	Sitting near the door in church	76
Feeling trapped at hairdresser, etc.	89	Focusing thoughts on something else	63
Increasing distance from home	87	Taking the dog, baby carriage, etc., along	62
Being at particular places in neighborhood	66	Being accompanied by a friend	60
Being in cloudy, depressing weather	56	Reassuring self	52
		Wearing sunglasses	36

Source. Adapted from Burns LE, Thorpe GL: "The Epidemiology of Fears and Phobias (With Particular Reference to the National Survey of Agoraphobics)." *Journal of International Medical Research* 5 (suppl): 1–7, 1977.

and dosages described for that condition. Exposure therapy is the most effective behavioral intervention and in its basic form consists of encouraging patients to gradually enter feared situations, such as a grocery store.

Generalized Anxiety Disorder

Patients with GAD worry excessively about life circumstances, such as their health, finances, social acceptance, job performance, and marital adjustment. Worry is central to the diagnosis. The criteria require that the individual have at least three of six symptoms: feeling restless or keyed up, being easily fatigued, having difficulty concentrating, being irritable, having muscle tension, or experiencing poor sleep. The symptoms must be present more days than not and cause clinically significant distress or impairment in social, occupational, or other important areas of functioning. The effects of a substance or a general medical condition should be ruled out as a cause of the symptoms. The condition must persist for 6 months or longer.

GAD has a lifetime prevalence of 4%–7% in the general population. Rates are higher among women, African Americans, and persons younger than 30 years. The disorder often has an onset during a patient's early 20s, but it can develop at any age. GAD usually is chronic, with symptoms that fluctuate in severity.

Frequent comorbidities include major depressive disorder and other anxiety disorders. Some patients use alcohol or drugs to control their symptoms, which can lead to a substance use disorder.

The differential diagnosis of GAD is similar to that for panic disorder. It is important to rule out drug-induced conditions such as caffeine intoxication, stimulant abuse, and alcohol, benzodiazepine, and sedative-hypnotic withdrawal. The mental status examination and patient history should cover the diagnostic possibilities of panic disorder, specific phobias, social anxiety disorder, obsessive-compulsive disorder, schizophrenia, and major depression.

Treatment of GAD usually involves CBT and medication. Relaxation training, rebreathing exercises, and meditation can be taught easily and may be effective. Several medications are FDA-approved to treat GAD, including the SSRIs paroxetine (20–50 mg/day) and escitalopram (10–20 mg/day); the SNRIs venlafaxine (75–225 mg/day) and duloxetine (60–120 mg/day); and the nonbenzodiazepine anxiolytic buspirone (10–40 mg/day). These drugs generally are well tolerated but take several weeks for the full effect to take place. Benzodiazepines are rapidly effective but can be habit-forming. Their use should be limited to short periods (e.g., weeks or months) when anxiety is severe. Hydroxyzine (25–50 mg/day) may be helpful for some patients and has the advantage of being relatively safe.

Clinical Points for Anxiety Disorders

- Separation anxiety disorder and selective mutism are disorders of children in most cases. Treatment necessarily involves the parents, along with medication.

- Mild cases of panic might respond to CBT, but many patients will need medication.
  - SSRIs are drugs of choice because of their effectiveness and tolerability. TCAs and MAOIs work well but are second-line treatments because of their many adverse effects and dangerousness in overdose.
- Gently encourage a patient with agoraphobia to get out and explore the world.
  - Progress will not occur unless the phobic patient confronts the feared places or situations. Some patients will need formal behavioral therapy.
  - Patients with anxiety disorders should minimize intake of caffeine, a known anxiogenic.
- Behavioral techniques (e.g., exposure, flooding, desensitization) will help most persons with social anxiety disorder and specific phobias.
  - Some people with a social phobia respond well to medication. SSRIs and venlafaxine are the medications of choice because of their effectiveness and tolerability.
- GAD might respond to simple behavioral techniques (e.g., relaxation training), but many patients will need medication.
  - Buspirone, venlafaxine, and the SSRIs paroxetine and escitalopram are effective FDA-approved treatments.
  - Benzodiazepines, when used, should be prescribed for a limited time (e.g., weeks or months). Hydroxyzine is a relatively benign alternative.

Further Reading

American Psychiatric Association: Practice guideline for the treatment of patients with panic disorder, second edition. Am J Psychiatry 166(suppl):5–68, 2009

Bandelow B, Michaelis S, Wedekind D: Treatment of anxiety disorders. Dialogues Clin Neurosci 19(2):93–107, 2017

Burns LE, Thorpe GL: The epidemiology of fears and phobias (with particular reference to the National Survey of Agoraphobics). J Int Med Res 5 (suppl 5):1–7, 1977

Liebowitz MR, Gelenberg AJ, Munjack D: Venlafaxine extended release vs placebo and paroxetine in social anxiety disorder. Arch Gen Psychiatry 62(2):190–198, 2005

Ravindran LN, Stein MB: The pharmacologic treatment of anxiety disorders: a review of progress. J Clin Psychiatry 71(7):839–854, 2010

Roberson-Nay R, Eaves LJ, Hettema JM, et al: Childhood separation anxiety disorder and adult onset panic attacks share a common genetic diathesis. Depress Anxiety 29(4):320–327, 2012

Schumacher J, Kristensen AS, Wendland JR, et al: The genetics of panic disorder. J Med Genet 48(6):361–368, 2011

Stein DJ, Hollander E, Rothbaum BO (eds): Textbook of Anxiety Disorders, 2nd Edition. Washington, DC, American Psychiatric Publishing, 2010

Chapter 7

Obsessive-Compulsive and Related Disorders

Obsessive-compulsive disorder (OCD) was previously classified with the anxiety disorders. In DSM-5, OCD forms the core of a new chapter that brings together related disorders (Table 7–1). Hoarding disorder and excoriation (skin-picking) disorder are new to DSM-5.

Obsessive-Compulsive Disorder

Obsessions and compulsions are the hallmarks of OCD. To receive the diagnosis, a person must have either obsessions or compulsions (most have both) that cause marked anxiety or distress and are time-consuming (more than 1 hour daily) or significantly interfere with the person's normal routine, occupational functioning, or usual social activities and relationships. The DSM-5 criteria for obsessive-compulsive disorder are shown in Box 7–1.

Box 7–1.   DSM-5 Criteria for Obsessive-
            Compulsive Disorder

A. Presence of obsessions, compulsions, or both:

Obsessions are defined by (1) and (2):

1. Recurrent and persistent thoughts, urges, or images that are experienced, at some time during the disturbance, as intrusive and unwanted, and that in most individuals cause marked anxiety or distress.
2. The individual attempts to ignore or suppress such thoughts, urges, or images, or to neutralize them with some other thought or action (i.e., by performing a compulsion).

Compulsions are defined by (1) and (2):

1. Repetitive behaviors (e.g., hand washing, ordering, checking) or mental acts (e.g., praying, counting, repeating

words silently) that the individual feels driven to perform in response to an obsession or according to rules that must be applied rigidly.

2. The behaviors or mental acts are aimed at preventing or reducing anxiety or distress, or preventing some dreaded event or situation; however, these behaviors or mental acts are not connected in a realistic way with what they are designed to neutralize or prevent, or are clearly excessive.

Note: Young children may not be able to articulate the aims of these behaviors or mental acts.

B. The obsessions or compulsions are time-consuming (e.g., take more than 1 hour per day) or cause clinically significant distress or impairment in social, occupational, or other important areas of functioning.

C. The obsessive-compulsive symptoms are not attributable to the physiological effects of a substance (e.g., a drug of abuse, a medication) or another medical condition.

D. The disturbance is not better explained by the symptoms of another mental disorder (e.g., excessive worries, as in generalized anxiety disorder; preoccupation with appearance, as in body dysmorphic disorder; difficulty discarding or parting with possessions, as in hoarding disorder; hair pulling, as in trichotillomania [hair-pulling disorder]; skin picking, as in excoriation [skin-picking] disorder; stereotypies, as in stereotypic movement disorder; ritualized eating behavior, as in eating disorders; preoccupation with substances or gambling, as in substance-related and addictive disorders; preoccupation with having an illness, as in illness anxiety disorder; sexual urges or fantasies, as in paraphilic disorders; impulses, as in disruptive, impulse-control, and conduct disorders; guilty ruminations, as in major depressive disorder; thought insertion or delusional preoccupations, as in schizophrenia spectrum and other psychotic disorders; or repetitive patterns of behavior, as in autism spectrum disorder).

Specify if:

With good or fair insight: The individual recognizes that obsessive-compulsive disorder beliefs are definitely or probably not true or that they may or may not be true.

With poor insight: The individual thinks obsessive-compulsive disorder beliefs are probably true.

With absent insight/delusional beliefs: The individual is completely convinced that obsessive-compulsive disorder beliefs are true.

Specify if:

Tic-related: The individual has a current or past history of a tic disorder.

TABLE 7–1. DSM-5 obsessive-compulsive and related disorders

Obsessive-compulsive disorder

Body dysmorphic disorder

Hoarding disorder

Trichotillomania (hair-pulling disorder)

Excoriation (skin-picking) disorder

Substance/medication-induced obsessive-compulsive and related disorder

Obsessive-compulsive and related disorder due to another medical condition

TABLE 7–2. Frequencies of common obsessions and compulsions in 560 patients with obsessive-compulsive disorder

Obsessions	%	Compulsions	%
Contamination	50	Checking	61
Pathological doubt	42	Washing	50
Somatic	33	Counting	36
Need for symmetry	32	Need to ask or confess	34
Aggressive impulse	31	Symmetry and precision	28
Sexual impulse	24	Hoarding	18
Multiple obsessions	72	Multiple compulsions	58

Source. Adapted from Rasmussen SA, Eisen JL: "Epidemiology and Clinical Features of Obsessive-Compulsive Disorder," in *Obsessive-Compulsive Disorders: Theory and Management*, 3rd Edition. Edited by Jenike MA, Baer L, Minichiello WE. St Louis, MO, CV Mosby, 1998, pp. 12–43.

Obsessions are recurrent and persistent ideas, thoughts, impulses, or images that are experienced as intrusive and inappropriate and cause marked anxiety or distress.

Compulsions are repetitive and intentional behaviors (or mental acts) designed to neutralize or reduce discomfort caused by an obsession, or to prevent a dreaded event or situation. The frequencies of common obsessions and compulsions are presented in Table 7–2.

In DSM-5, OCD is subtyped according to the patient's degree of current insight (good or fair, poor, absent/delusional), as well as whether the disorder is related to tics. Poor insight tends to be associated with poor outcome. The *tic-related* subtype is highly familial and is associated with a better response when an antipsychotic is added to a selective serotonin reuptake inhibitor (SSRI).

Epidemiology and Clinical Findings

OCD typically begins in the late teens or early 20s. Most persons with the disorder will have developed it by age 30 years. The disorder has a lifetime prevalence of 2%–3% in the general population. Men and women are equally likely to develop OCD, but men tend to have an earlier onset. In a study of 250 OCD patients, 85% had a chronic course, 10% a progressive or deteriorating course, and 2% an episodic course with periods of remission. Future studies likely will show more favorable outcomes, given that effective treatments are now available.

Mild symptoms and good premorbid adjustment are associated with better outcome. Early onset and the presence of a personality disorder have been associated with poor outcome. Patients typically report that their OCD symptoms are worse when they are depressed or experiencing stressful situations. Recurrent episodes of major depressive disorder occur in 70%–80% of OCD patients.

Etiology and Pathophysiology

OCD has a considerable genetic component based on family and twin studies and is linked with Tourette's disorder. OCD might be considered a neuropsychiatric disorder because it occurs more often in persons with epilepsy, Sydenham's chorea, and Huntington's chorea and has been linked to birth injuries and abnormal electroencephalographic findings. One particular type of OCD, PANDAS (pediatric autoimmune neuropsychiatric disorders associated with streptococcal infections), has been identified in children who have had a group A β-streptococcal infection. These children not only develop obsessions and compulsions but also have emotional lability, separation anxiety, and tics.

The neurotransmitter serotonin has been the focus of great interest, perhaps because antidepressant drugs that block its reuptake—SSRIs—are effective in treating OCD, whereas other antidepressants are not effective. Other evidence supporting the "serotonin hypothesis" is indirect but is consistent with the view that either levels of the neurotransmitter are disturbed or the number or function of serotonin receptors is altered in OCD patients.

Imaging studies have shown basal ganglia involvement in some persons with OCD. Studies using positron emission tomography (PET) or single-photon emission computed tomography (SPECT) scanning in OCD patients have found increased glucose metabolism in the caudate nuclei and the orbital cortex of the frontal lobes—abnormalities that partially reverse with treatment. Possibly basal ganglia dysfunction leads to the complex motor processes involved in OCD, whereas the prefrontal hyperactivity might be related to the tendency to worry and plan excessively.

Differential Diagnosis

The differential diagnosis includes schizophrenia, major depressive disorder, posttraumatic stress disorder, hypochondriasis, anorexia nervosa, Tourette's disorder, and obsessive-compulsive personality disorder. Obsessive-compulsive personality disorder is characterized by perfectionism, orderliness, and obstinacy, while OCD patients are more likely to have dependent, avoidant, or passive-aggressive personality traits.

Clinical Management

Treating OCD usually involves medication combined with cognitive-behavioral therapy (CBT), mainly exposure paired with response prevention. For example, a patient might be exposed to a dreaded situation, event, or stimulus by techniques such as imaginal exposure, systematic desensitization, and flooding and then prevented from carrying out the compulsive behavior that usually results. A compulsive washer might be asked to handle "contaminated" objects (e.g., a dirty tissue) and then be prevented from washing his or her hands.

Several SSRIs are FDA-approved for treating OCD, including fluoxetine, fluvoxamine, paroxetine, and sertraline. Clomipramine, a tricyclic antidepressant that is a relatively specific serotonin reuptake blocker, also is approved for treating OCD. Because of its many adverse effects, clomipramine is used less frequently than the SSRIs.

Typically, higher dosages of SSRIs are needed to treat OCD than those used to treat major depressive disorder, and response often is delayed. For that reason, initiate relatively lengthy trials (i.e., 12–16 weeks) for patients. Adding an antipsychotic might boost the likelihood of response in patients whose disorder does not respond to SSRIs.

Some patients with treatment-refractory illness who undergo specific psychosurgical procedures (e.g., cingulotomy, deep brain stimulation) can experience benefit. However, these options are not widely available.

Body Dysmorphic Disorder

The patient with body dysmorphic disorder (BDD), formerly called *dysmorphophobia*, is preoccupied with an imagined defect or flaws in physical appearance that cannot be observed or appear slight to others. For this reason, BDD sometimes is referred to as "the disease of imagined ugliness." A specifier is available for those individuals with *muscle dysmorphia*, a condition found almost exclusively in men who believe they are insufficiently muscular.

BDD has an estimated prevalence of 1%–3% in the general population and is equally common among men and women. Onset occurs in adolescence or early adulthood. BDD tends to be chronic, but it fluctuates in intensity and severity; few individuals experience remission. The disorder can significantly impair the person's social and occupational functioning. Nearly all attribute their disability to the embarrassment associated with their imagined defect. Patients who are concerned about their facial appearance sometimes undergo repeated plastic surgery procedures but rarely are satisfied with the results.

Some individuals with BDD are delusional and cannot be persuaded that their beliefs about their appearance are false. In these cases, the patient should receive a diagnosis of BDD "with absent insight/delusional beliefs," and not delusional disorder.

BDD is treated with SSRIs and CBT. A positive response to medication means that the patient is less distressed and preoccupied by his or her thoughts about the "defect" and reports improved social and occupational functioning. In delusional forms of BDD, a second-generation antipsychotic (e.g., olanzapine, risperidone) added to the SSRI may boost response. With CBT, patients are encouraged to reassess their distorted beliefs about the "defect" and to modify behaviors that appear to encourage their preoccupation, such as mirror gazing.

Hoarding Disorder

Hoarding disorder is new to DSM-5 and is characterized by collecting objects that are of limited value or are worthless and being unable to discard them. Many people refer to this as the "pack rat" syndrome, although patients are more likely to think of themselves as collectors. Significant hoarding has been shown to occur in up to 5% of the general population.

The central feature of hoarding disorder is the intention to save possessions. Clutter results from purposeful saving and reluctance to discard items because they have sentimental significance, are potentially useful, or have intrinsic aesthetic value. Frequently hoarded items include clothes, newspapers, and magazines.

Several other conditions can lead to clutter and difficulty discarding possessions and should be ruled out. For example, hoarding behaviors can occur in people with lesions in the anterior ventromedial prefrontal and cingulate cortices. Also, individuals with Prader-Willi syndrome—a rare genetic disorder associated with short stature, hyperphagia, insatiability, and food-seeking behavior—display hoarding behavior, associated mostly with food but with nonfood items as well.

Hoarding also can occur in individuals with severe dementia, which appears to stem from significant cognitive deterioration, not an attachment to objects. Hoarding has been described in patients with schizophrenia, but it also does not appear in that context to be motivated by an attachment to objects. OCD is the condition most closely associated with hoarding, and up to 30% of individuals with the disorder will show some degree of hoarding behavior.

Treating hoarding disorder is challenging, with few patients responding well to either SSRIs or CBT. For some, the best option might be to hire a personal organizer or a trusted friend or relative who can help with cleaning up the person's home. Consistent monitoring afterwards can help prevent re-accumulation.

Trichotillomania (Hair-Pulling Disorder)

Trichotillomania (hair-pulling disorder) is characterized by recurrent pulling out of one's hair that results in noticeable hair loss. Affected individuals usually experience an increasing sense of tension before engaging in the behavior and pleasure, gratification, or relief when pulling out the hair. Persons with trichotillomania usually report substantial subjective distress or develop other evidence of impairment.

The disorder generally is chronic, although it might wax and wane in severity. It can affect any site where hair grows, including the scalp, eyelids, eyebrows, body, and axillary and pubic regions. Most hair pullers are female, and they typically report onset during childhood. Surveys show that it affects 1%–4% of adolescents and college students. Compulsive hair pullers frequently have comorbid mood and anxiety disorders.

The diagnosis is made easily after other diagnoses and medical conditions have been ruled out. Most patients have no obvious balding, but instead have small bald spots or patches or missing eyebrows and eyelashes.

Treatment consists of medication and *habit reversal therapy*, often in combination. Patients learn to identify when their hair pulling occurs (it often is automatic) and to substitute a benign behavior such as squeezing a ball. Some patients benefit from learning to apply barriers to prevent hair pulling, such as wearing gloves or a hat.

SSRIs or clomipramine is probably the most frequently prescribed medication for trichotillomania and might help reduce urges to pull. A recent study suggested that the glutamate modulator *N*-acetylcysteine might be effective.

Excoriation (Skin-Picking) Disorder

Excoriation (skin-picking) disorder is new to DSM-5. People with this disorder repetitively and compulsively pick at their skin, leading to tissue damage. Skin picking is relatively common, occurring in approximately 1%–5% of the general population. Often considered chronic, the disorder fluctuates in intensity and severity. The face is the most common site of picking; other areas, such as hands, fingers, torso, arms, and legs, also are common targets. Picking could result in significant tissue damage and may lead to medical complications such as localized infections or septicemia. In rare cases, stimulants can cause skin picking behaviors; therefore, rule out stimulant use. Also rule out dermatological conditions such as scabies, atopic dermatitis, psoriasis, and blistering skin disorders. Treatment is not well established but often consists of the same elements as trichotillomania treatment: SSRIs to lessen urges, and habit reversal techniques to address the skin picking.

Clinical Points for Obsessive-Compulsive and Related Disorders

- Educate the patient about his or her OCD:

  - To reduce feelings of isolation, fear, and confusion.

  - To reassure worried patients that people with OCD rarely act on their frightening or violent obsessions.

  - To point out the "up" side of OCD: that people with the disorder tend to be conscientious, dependable, and likeable.

- Establish an empathic relationship.

  - Do not tell patients to stop their rituals; they can't. That's why they are seeking help.

  - Explain that talking about their obsessions and compulsions will not make them worse.

- Patients generally do best with both medication and behavioral therapy.

  - Clomipramine and SSRIs usually are effective. With SSRIs, higher dosages will be needed than those used to treat depression.

  - The lag time to improvement with medication is months, not weeks as in the treatment of depression.

- Body dysmorphic disorder often responds well to SSRIs.

  - Even delusional forms of the disorder tend not to require antipsychotic medication.

- With hoarding disorder, think "outside the box."

  - Medication and psychotherapy do not appear to be especially helpful.

  - Some patients benefit from hiring a personal organizer to help clear out the house, if feasible.

- Trichotillomania probably responds best to behavioral therapy.

  - Habit reversal methods have shown benefit.

  - SSRIs or clomipramine could reduce the urge to pull, but response to these drugs is inconsistent.

  - For patients with extensive hair loss, wigs and other forms of hair replacement might be the most sensible solution to restore self-esteem and boost morale.

- Because excoriation disorder strongly resembles trichotillomania, habit reversal techniques could be beneficial.

Further Reading

Browne HA, Hansen SN, Buxbaum JD, et al: Familial clustering of tic disorders and obsessive-compulsive disorder. JAMA Psychiatry 72(4):359–366, 2015

Grant JE, Stein DJ, Woods DW, Keuthen NJ: Trichotillomania, Skin Picking, and Other Body-Focused Repetitive Behaviors. Washington, DC, American Psychiatric Publishing, 2012

Koran LM, Hanna GL, Hollander E, et al; American Psychiatric Association: Practice guideline for the treatment of patients with obsessive-compulsive disorder. Am J Psychiatry 164 (7, suppl):5–53, 2007

Phillips KA, Didie ER, Feusner J, Wilhelm S: Body dysmorphic disorder: treating an underrecognized disorder. Am J Psychiatry 165(9):1111–1118, 2008

Rasmussen SA, Eisen JL: Epidemiology and clinical features of obsessive-compulsive disorder, in Obsessive-Compulsive Disorders: Theory and Management, 3rd Edition. Edited by Jenike MA, Baer L, Minichiello WE. St Louis, MO, CV Mosby, 1998, pp 12–43

Rück C, Karlsson A, Steele JD, et al: Capsulotomy for obsessive-compulsive disorder: long-term follow-up of 25 patients. Arch Gen Psychiatry 65(8):914–921, 2008

Schwartz JM, Stoessel PW, Baxter LR Jr, et al: Systematic changes in cerebral glucose metabolic rate after successful behavior modification treatment of obsessive-compulsive disorder. Arch Gen Psychiatry 53(2):109–113, 1996

Simpson HB, Foa EB, Liebowitz MR, et al: A randomized, controlled trial of cognitive-behavioral therapy for augmenting pharmacotherapy in obsessive-compulsive disorder. Am J Psychiatry 165(5):621–630, 2008

Skoog G, Skoog I: A 40-year follow-up of patients with obsessive-compulsive disorder [see comments]. Arch Gen Psychiatry 56(2):121–127, 1999

Chapter 8

Trauma- and Stressor-Related Disorders

Trauma- and stressor-related disorders is a new diagnostic class in DSM-5 that brings together acute stress disorder, posttraumatic stress disorder (PTSD), reactive attachment disorder, disinhibited social engagement disorder (DSED), and adjustment disorders. Disorders in this class each result from exposure to traumatic or stressful situations or events explicitly described in the diagnostic criteria. These are among the few conditions in DSM-5 that have a direct cause-and-effect relationship. The DSM-5 trauma- and stressor-related disorders are listed in Table 8–1.

Reactive Attachment Disorder and Disinhibited Social Engagement Disorder

Reactive attachment disorder and DSED are characterized by disturbances in attachment behaviors that normally occur between a child and caregiver (usually a parent) and result from parental neglect or abuse.

Reactive attachment disorder is rare in clinical settings, and even among severely neglected children the disorder is uncommon, occurring in less than 10% of such children. With reactive attachment disorder, attachment is either absent or underdeveloped. The disorder might be associated with signs of severe neglect (e.g., malnutrition, poor hygiene) and may be accompanied by delays in speaking and cognitive development.

Children with this condition show little responsiveness to others and make scant effort to obtain comfort, support, nurturance, or protection from caregivers. In DSM-5, the child must have reached a developmental age of 9 months, which ensures that reactive attachment disorder is not diagnosed in

TABLE 8–1. DSM-5 trauma- and stressor-related disorders

Reactive attachment disorder

Disinhibited social engagement disorder

Posttraumatic stress disorder

Acute stress disorder

Adjustment disorders

children who are developmentally incapable of having a focused attachment.

The differential diagnosis includes autism spectrum disorder. The disorders can be distinguished on the basis of developmental histories of neglect, the presence of restricted interests or ritualized behaviors, specific deficits in social communication, and the presence of selective attachment behaviors.

It is crucial that children with reactive attachment disorder be removed from the home in which there is abuse or neglect and be placed in foster care. The child must be provided with a secure and stable living situation with a nurturing caregiver and access to appropriate medical care. Treatment includes both individual psychotherapy and family therapy to address the disturbed emotions and relationships.

Disinhibited social engagement disorder is new to DSM-5. Unlike reactive attachment disorder, its essential feature is a pattern of behavior that involves inappropriate and overly familiar behavior with relative strangers, therefore violating the social boundaries of the culture. The diagnosis requires the presence of two or more of four examples of disinhibited behavior. These include reduced (or absent) reticence with unfamiliar adults, overly familiar behavior, diminished or absent checking back, and willingness to go away with an unfamiliar adult with little or no hesitation. The prevalence of DSED is unknown, but its occurrence in foster care or shared residential facilities might be as high as 20%.

DSED is associated with cognitive and language delays, stereotypies, and other signs of severe neglect, including malnutrition and poor hygiene. Signs of the disorder could persist even when the neglect is no longer present. Treatment tends to be directed at improving relatedness and interpersonal functioning.

Posttraumatic Stress Disorder

PTSD occurs in individuals who have been exposed to actual or threatened death, serious physical injury, or sexual violence. The event typically is outside the range of normal human experience. Examples of such events include combat, physical assault, rape, and disasters (e.g., home fires). The DSM-5 criteria for PTSD are shown in Box 8–1.

Two subtypes are specified in DSM-5: *with dissociative symptoms*, when derealization or depersonalization is present, and *with delayed expression*, if onset is delayed until at least 6 months after the traumatic event.

Box 8–1.   DSM-5 Criteria for Posttraumatic Stress Disorder

Note: The following criteria apply to adults, adolescents, and children older than 6 years. For children 6 years and younger, see corresponding criteria in DSM-5.

A. Exposure to actual or threatened death, serious injury, or sexual violence in one (or more) of the following ways:

1. Directly experiencing the traumatic event(s).

2. Witnessing, in person, the event(s) as it occurred to others.

3. Learning that the traumatic event(s) occurred to a close family member or close friend. In cases of actual or threatened death of a family member or friend, the event(s) must have been violent or accidental.

4. Experiencing repeated or extreme exposure to aversive details of the traumatic event(s) (e.g., first responders collecting human remains; police officers repeatedly exposed to details of child abuse).

    Note: Criterion A4 does not apply to exposure through electronic media, television, movies, or pictures, unless this exposure is work related.

B. Presence of one (or more) of the following intrusion symptoms associated with the traumatic event(s), beginning after the traumatic event(s) occurred:

1. Recurrent, involuntary, and intrusive distressing memories of the traumatic event(s).

    Note: In children older than 6 years, repetitive play may occur in which themes or aspects of the traumatic event(s) are expressed.

2. Recurrent distressing dreams in which the content and/or affect of the dream are related to the traumatic event(s).

Note: In children, there may be frightening dreams without recognizable content.

3. Dissociative reactions (e.g., flashbacks) in which the individual feels or acts as if the traumatic event(s) were recurring. (Such reactions may occur on a continuum, with the most extreme expression being a complete loss of awareness of present surroundings.)

Note: In children, trauma-specific reenactment may occur in play.

4. Intense or prolonged psychological distress at exposure to internal or external cues that symbolize or resemble an aspect of the traumatic event(s).

5. Marked physiological reactions to internal or external cues that symbolize or resemble an aspect of the traumatic event(s).

C. Persistent avoidance of stimuli associated with the traumatic event(s), beginning after the traumatic event(s) occurred, as evidenced by one or both of the following:

1. Avoidance of or efforts to avoid distressing memories, thoughts, or feelings about or closely associated with the traumatic event(s).

2. Avoidance of or efforts to avoid external reminders (people, places, conversations, activities, objects, situations) that arouse distressing memories, thoughts, or feelings about or closely associated with the traumatic event(s).

D. Negative alterations in cognitions and mood associated with the traumatic event(s), beginning or worsening after the traumatic event(s) occurred, as evidenced by two (or more) of the following:

1. Inability to remember an important aspect of the traumatic event(s) (typically due to dissociative amnesia and not to other factors such as head injury, alcohol, or drugs).

2. Persistent and exaggerated negative beliefs or expectations about oneself, others, or the world (e.g., "I am bad," "No one can be trusted," "The world is completely dangerous," "My whole nervous system is permanently ruined").

3. Persistent, distorted cognitions about the cause or consequences of the traumatic event(s) that lead the individual to blame himself/herself or others.

4. Persistent negative emotional state (e.g., fear, horror, anger, guilt, or shame).

5. Markedly diminished interest or participation in significant activities.
6. Feelings of detachment or estrangement from others.
7. Persistent inability to experience positive emotions (e.g., inability to experience happiness, satisfaction, or loving feelings).

E. Marked alterations in arousal and reactivity associated with the traumatic event(s), beginning or worsening after the traumatic event(s) occurred, as evidenced by two (or more) of the following:

1. Irritable behavior and angry outbursts (with little or no provocation) typically expressed as verbal or physical aggression toward people or objects.
2. Reckless or self-destructive behavior.
3. Hypervigilance.
4. Exaggerated startle response.
5. Problems with concentration.
6. Sleep disturbance (e.g., difficulty falling or staying asleep or restless sleep).

F. Duration of the disturbance (Criteria B, C, D, and E) is more than 1 month.

G. The disturbance causes clinically significant distress or impairment in social, occupational, or other important areas of functioning.

H. The disturbance is not attributable to the physiological effects of a substance (e.g., medication, alcohol) or another medical condition.

Epidemiology and Clinical Findings

PTSD has a prevalence of nearly 7% in the general population. Most men with the disorder have experienced combat. For women, the most frequent precipitating event is a physical assault or rape. The disorder can occur at any age, and even young children can develop the disorder.

PTSD generally begins soon after the stressor is experienced, but its onset may be delayed for months or years. The disorder is chronic for many, but symptoms fluctuate and typically worsen during stressful periods. Rapid onset of symptoms, good premorbid functioning, strong social support, and the absence of psychiatric or medical comorbidity are factors associated with a good outcome. Many patients with PTSD have comorbid psychiatric disorders such as major depressive disorder, anxiety disorders, or alcohol or drug use disorders.

Etiology and Pathophysiology

The major etiological factor leading to PTSD is a traumatic event, which must be severe enough to be outside the range of normal human experience. Business losses, marital conflicts, and death of a loved one are *not* considered stressors that cause PTSD. Research shows that the more severe the trauma, the greater the risk of developing PTSD.

A person's age, history of emotional disturbance, level of social support, and proximity to the stressor are all factors that affect the likelihood of developing PTSD. Eighty percent of young children who sustain burn injuries show symptoms of posttraumatic stress 1–2 years after the injury, but only 30% of adults who sustain similar injuries do so. Those who have received psychiatric treatment in the past are more likely to develop PTSD, presumably because the previous illness reflects the person's greater vulnerability to stress. Persons with adequate social support are less likely to develop PTSD than those with poor support.

Research suggests that the sustained levels of high emotional arousal can lead to dysregulation of the hypothalamic-pituitary-adrenal axis. The noradrenergic and serotonergic pathways in the central nervous system also have been implicated in the genesis of PTSD. Brain imaging is helping researchers understand the underlying neurobiology of PTSD. Reduced hippocampal volume and increased metabolic activity in limbic regions, particularly the amygdala, are the most replicated findings. These findings may help to explain the role of disturbed emotional memory in PTSD.

Differential Diagnosis

The differential diagnosis of PTSD includes major depressive disorder, adjustment disorder, panic disorder, generalized anxiety disorder, acute stress disorder, obsessive-compulsive disorder, depersonalization/derealization disorder, factitious disorder, or malingering. In some cases, a physical injury might have occurred during the traumatic event, necessitating a physical and neurological examination.

Clinical Management

The selective serotonin reuptake inhibitors (SSRIs) paroxetine (20–50 mg/day) and sertraline (50–200 mg/day) are FDA-approved for treating PTSD, although other SSRIs likely are effective. These drugs help to decrease depressive symptoms, reduce intrusive symptoms such as nightmares and flashbacks, and normalize sleep. The serotonin-norepinephrine reuptake inhibitor venlafaxine also appears to be effective. Benzodiazepines might help reduce anxiety but should be used for short-term treatment (e.g., days to weeks) because they could be habit-forming. The α_1-adrenergic antagonist prazosin (up to 10 mg/day) appears to be effective in alleviating the intractable nightmares that some PTSD patients report.

Establishing a sense of safety and separation from the trauma is an important first step when treating PTSD. Cultivating a therapeutic working relationship requires time for the patient to develop trust. Cognitive-behavioral therapy (CBT) is effective in reducing PTSD symptoms by providing patients skills to control anxiety and to counter dysfunctional thoughts (e.g., "I deserved to be raped"). Controlled exposure to cues associated with the trauma could be helpful in decreasing avoidance. Group therapy and family therapy also are useful and have been widely recommended for combat veterans. Some recommend eye movement desensitization and reprocessing (EMDR) therapy, but research suggests that its efficacy is driven by its exposure component.

Acute Stress Disorder

Acute stress disorder occurs in some individuals after a traumatic experience and is considered a precursor to PTSD. By definition, the individual must have 9 or more of 14 symptoms from five categories: intrusion symptoms, negative mood, dissociative symptoms, avoidance symptoms, and arousal symptoms. The symptoms must cause clinically significant difficulties in functioning and last from 3 days up to 1 month after trauma exposure. The DSM-5 criteria for acute stress disorder are shown in Box 8–2.

Box 8–2.   DSM-5 Criteria for Acute Stress Disorder

A. Exposure to actual or threatened death, serious injury, or sexual violation in one (or more) of the following ways:

1. Directly experiencing the traumatic event(s).
2. Witnessing, in person, the event(s) as it occurred to others.
3. Learning that the event(s) occurred to a close family member or close friend. **Note:** In cases of actual or threatened

death of a family member or friend, the event(s) must have been violent or accidental.

4. Experiencing repeated or extreme exposure to aversive details of the traumatic event(s) (e.g., first responders collecting human remains, police officers repeatedly exposed to details of child abuse).

   Note: This does not apply to exposure through electronic media, television, movies, or pictures, unless this exposure is work related.

B. Presence of nine (or more) of the following symptoms from any of the five categories of intrusion, negative mood, dissociation, avoidance, and arousal, beginning or worsening after the traumatic event(s) occurred:

Intrusion Symptoms

1. Recurrent, involuntary, and intrusive distressing memories of the traumatic event(s). Note: In children, repetitive play may occur in which themes or aspects of the traumatic event(s) are expressed.

2. Recurrent distressing dreams in which the content and/or affect of the dream are related to the event(s). Note: In children, there may be frightening dreams without recognizable content.

3. Dissociative reactions (e.g., flashbacks) in which the individual feels or acts as if the traumatic event(s) were recurring. (Such reactions may occur on a continuum, with the most extreme expression being a complete loss of awareness of present surroundings.) Note: In children, trauma-specific reenactment may occur in play.

4. Intense or prolonged psychological distress or marked physiological reactions in response to internal or external cues that symbolize or resemble an aspect of the traumatic event(s).

Negative Mood

5. Persistent inability to experience positive emotions (e.g., inability to experience happiness, satisfaction, or loving feelings).

Dissociative Symptoms

6. An altered sense of the reality of one's surroundings or oneself (e.g., seeing oneself from another's perspective, being in a daze, time slowing).

7. Inability to remember an important aspect of the traumatic event(s) (typically due to dissociative amnesia and not to other factors such as head injury, alcohol, or drugs).

Avoidance Symptoms

8. Efforts to avoid distressing memories, thoughts, or feelings about or closely associated with the traumatic event(s).
9. Efforts to avoid external reminders (people, places, conversations, activities, objects, situations) that arouse distressing memories, thoughts, or feelings about or closely associated with the traumatic event(s).

Arousal Symptoms

10. Sleep disturbance (e.g., difficulty falling or staying asleep, restless sleep).
11. Irritable behavior and angry outbursts (with little or no provocation), typically expressed as verbal or physical aggression toward people or objects.
12. Hypervigilance.
13. Problems with concentration.
14. Exaggerated startle response.

C. Duration of the disturbance (symptoms in Criterion B) is 3 days to 1 month after trauma exposure.

Note: Symptoms typically begin immediately after the trauma, but persistence for at least 3 days and up to a month is needed to meet disorder criteria.

D. The disturbance causes clinically significant distress or impairment in social, occupational, or other important areas of functioning.
E. The disturbance is not attributable to the physiological effects of a substance (e.g., medication or alcohol) or another medical condition (e.g., mild traumatic brain injury) and is not better explained by brief psychotic disorder.

Acute stress disorder occurs in less than 20% of individuals after a traumatic event. Higher rates have been reported after interpersonal traumatic events such as an assault, rape, or witnessing a mass shooting. Women seem to be at greater risk for developing acute stress disorder.

The differential diagnosis of acute stress disorder includes PTSD, brief psychotic disorder, a dissociative disorder, or adjustment disorder.

CBT involving exposure and anxiety management (e.g., relaxation training, re-breathing) has been shown to help prevent the progression to full-blown PTSD. When anxiety is severe, a brief course of a benzodiazepine may be helpful.

Adjustment Disorders

Adjustment disorders lead to emotional or behavioral symptoms arising from a person's response to a stressful event, such as job loss, marital problems, or financial distress. By definition, the symptoms causing an adjustment disorder must arise within 3 months of a stressor and must be clinically significant. The symptoms cannot merely represent exacerbation of a preexisting disorder, and they cannot be represented by normal bereavement. Furthermore, the maladaptive reaction cannot persist for more than 6 months after the termination of the stressor or its consequences.

Epidemiology and Clinical Findings

Adjustment disorders are common, and their prevalence in psychiatric clinics and hospitals is estimated to range from 5% to 20% of individuals seeking care. The diagnosis is more common in women. Adjustment disorders can occur at any age, but the mean age at diagnosis tends to be in the mid-20s to early 30s. Common symptoms in adolescents include behavioral changes or acting out. Adults typically develop mood or anxiety symptoms.

Different subtypes of adjustment disorder reflect the varied symptoms that can occur in response to a stressor:

- *Depressed mood:* dysphoria, tearfulness, hopelessness
- *Anxiety:* psychic anxiety, palpitations, jitteriness, hyperventilation
- *Conduct disturbance:* violating the rights of others or disregarding age-appropriate societal norms and rules (e.g., vandalism, reckless driving, fighting)
- *Mixed disturbance of emotions and conduct:* emotional symptoms, such as depression or anxiety, in addition to a behavioral disturbance
- *Unspecified:* for example, a person who has developed difficulty functioning at work

Differential Diagnosis

In making a diagnosis of adjustment disorder, the crucial question is *"What is the patient having trouble adjusting to?"* Without a stressor, there is no adjustment disorder. Yet even when a stressor exists, other mental disorders need to be ruled out as the cause of the symptoms, and the stressor cannot represent normal bereavement. A person who experiences an important stressor (e.g., recent marital separation) and develops depressed mood receives a diagnosis of adjustment disorder *only* when his or her symptoms do not meet criteria for major depressive disorder.

The differential diagnosis includes mood disorders (e.g., major depressive disorder), anxiety disorders (e.g., panic disorder, generalized anxiety disorder), and conduct disorder in a child or adolescent. Consider personality disorders, because they are frequently associated with mood instability and behavior problems.

Clinical Management

Supportive psychotherapy probably is the most widely used treatment for adjustment disorders. A therapist can help the patient adapt to the stressor when it is ongoing or to better understand the stressor once it has passed. Group psychotherapy can provide a supportive atmosphere for persons who have experienced similar stressors, such as those who have received a diagnosis of breast cancer.

Prescribe medications on the basis of the patient's symptoms. For example, a patient with initial insomnia might benefit from a hypnotic (e.g., zolpidem, 5–10 mg at bedtime) for a few days. A patient experiencing anxiety may benefit from a brief course (e.g., days to weeks) of a benzodiazepine. If the disorder persists, reconsider the diagnosis. At some point, an adjustment disorder with depressed mood, for example, may develop into major depressive disorder, which would respond best to antidepressant medication.

Clinical Points for Trauma- and Stressor-Related Disorders

- Reactive attachment disorder and DSED result from abuse or neglectful care. In many cases the best response is to remove the child from the home and place him or her in a more nurturing environment.

- PTSD tends to be chronic, but many patients will benefit from a combination of medication and cognitive-behavioral therapy.

- Paroxetine and sertraline are FDA-approved for treating PTSD. Other SSRIs probably are effective as well.

- Prazosin may be effective in treating disturbing dreams and nightmares.

- Many patients with PTSD will benefit from the mutual support found in group therapy.

- Group therapy has become especially popular with veterans. Most veterans' organizations can offer help in finding a local group.

- Adjustment disorders can evolve into other, better defined disorders, such as major depressive disorder; therefore, be alert to changes in mental status and the evolution of symptoms.

- Most adjustment disorders are transient. Time and supportive therapy usually are all that is needed.

- Psychotropic medication taken short-term (i.e., days to weeks) target the predominant symptoms.

  - Hypnotics (e.g., zolpidem, 5–10 mg at bedtime) for those with insomnia.

  - Benzodiazepines (e.g., lorazepam, 0.5–2.0 mg twice daily) for those with anxiety.

  - If long-term treatment is needed, the patient might have another disorder (e.g., major depressive disorder) that will need to be diagnosed and treated.

Further Reading

Andreasen NC, Wasek P: Adjustment disorders in adolescents and adults. Arch Gen Psychiatry 37(10):1166–1170, 1980

Bryant RA, Creamer M, O'Donnell ML, et al: A multisite study of the capacity of acute stress disorder diagnosis to predict posttraumatic stress disorder. J Clin Psychiatry 69(6):923–929, 2008

Friedman MJ, Keane TM, Resick PA: Handbook of PTSD: Science and Practice, 2nd Edition. New York, Guilford, 2014

Heim C, Nemeroff CB: Neurobiology of posttraumatic stress disorder. CNS Spectr 14(1) (suppl 1):13–24, 2009

Jones R, Yates WR, Zhou MH: Readmission rates for adjustment disorders: comparison with other mood disorders. J Affect Disord 71(1–3):199–203, 2002

Mohamed S, Rosenheck RA: Pharmacotherapy of PTSD in the U.S. Department of Veterans Affairs: diagnostic- and symptom-guided drug selection. J Clin Psychiatry 69(6):959–965, 2008

North CS, Pfefferbaum B, Tivis L, et al: The course of posttraumatic stress disorder in a follow-up study of survivors of the Oklahoma City bombing. Ann Clin Psychiatry 16(4):209–215, 2004

Pelkonen M, Marttunen M, Henriksson M, Lönnqvist J: Adolescent adjustment disorder: precipitant stressors and distress symptoms of 89 outpatients. Eur Psychiatry 22(5):288–295, 2007

Raskind MA, Peskind ER, Hoff DJ, et al: A parallel group placebo controlled study of prazosin for trauma nightmares and sleep disturbance in combat veterans with post-traumatic stress disorder. Biol Psychiatry 61(8):928–934, 2007

Stein DJ, Hollander E, Rothbaum BO (eds): Textbook of Anxiety Disorders, 2nd Edition. Washington, DC, American Psychiatric Publishing, 2010

Ursano RJ, Bell C, Eth S, et al; Work Group on ASD and PTSD; Steering Committee on Practice Guidelines: Practice guideline for the treatment of patients with acute stress disorder and posttraumatic stress disorder. Am J Psychiatry 161 (11, suppl):3–31, 2004

Chapter 9

Dissociative Disorders

The hallmark of dissociative disorders is a disturbance of or alteration in the normally well-integrated functions of identity, memory, and consciousness. DSM-5 dissociative disorders are listed in Table 9–1.

Dissociation occurs along a spectrum. At the milder end, dissociation is a common and normal part of human consciousness. For example, most people have had the experience of driving somewhere and not remembering portions of the trip ("highway hypnosis"). In some people, however, the dissociative process becomes distorted and actively interferes with one's functioning, causing distress and disability. Symptoms can be experienced as unwanted intrusions into awareness and behavior with accompanying loss of continuity in subjective experience, or as an inability to access information or control mental functions that are amenable to access or control.

Dissociative Identity Disorder

Dissociative identity disorder (DID), formerly recognized as *multiple personality disorder*, is characterized by the presence of two or more distinct personality states, which in some cultures may be likened to possession (see Box 9–1). There is a marked discontinuity in sense of self and sense of agency, accompanied by related alterations in affect, behavior, consciousness, memory, perception, cognition, and/or sensory-motor functioning, as observed by others or reported by oneself.

Box 9–1. DSM-5 Criteria for Dissociative Identity Disorder

A. Disruption of identity characterized by two or more distinct personality states, which may be described in some cultures as an experience of possession. The disruption in identity involves marked discontinuity in sense of self and sense of agency, accompanied by related alterations in affect, behavior, consciousness, memory, perception, cognition, and/or sensory-motor functioning. These signs and symptoms may be observed by others or reported by the individual.

B. Recurrent gaps in the recall of everyday events, important personal information, and/or traumatic events that are inconsistent with ordinary forgetting.

C. The symptoms cause clinically significant distress or impairment in social, occupational, or other important areas of functioning.

D. The disturbance is not a normal part of a broadly accepted cultural or religious practice.

Note: In children, the symptoms are not better explained by imaginary playmates or other fantasy play.

E. The symptoms are not attributable to the physiological effects of a substance (e.g., blackouts or chaotic behavior during alcohol intoxication) or another medical condition (e.g., complex partial seizures).

DID has a prevalence of approximately 1.5% in the general population and is fairly common (5%–15%) in inpatient and outpatient psychiatric settings. The disorder was once thought to be rare, and the apparent increase in frequency has led some to question whether well-meaning therapists have unknowingly induced the disorder through suggestion and the process of hypnosis.

Most individuals diagnosed with DID are women. The disorder has a childhood onset, usually before age 9 years, and often is chronic. The most common symptoms reported by patients are listed in Table 9–2.

Some experts hypothesize that DID results from severe physical and sexual abuse during childhood. They believe that the disorder results from self-induced hypnosis, used by the individual to cope with abuse, emotional maltreatment, or neglect.

Similar to persons with posttraumatic stress disorder (PTSD), DID patients have smaller hippocampal and amygdalar volumes, suggesting that early traumatic experiences might affect neural circuitry in brain regions associated with memory.

Patients with DID often have unexplained physical complaints and symptoms that fulfill criteria for somatic symptom disorder. Headaches and amnesia ("losing time") are

TABLE 9–1. DSM-5 dissociative disorders

Dissociative identity disorder

Dissociative amnesia

Depersonalization/derealization disorder

TABLE 9–2. Common symptoms of dissociative identity disorder and characteristics of alternate personalities ("alters") (based on sample of 50 patients)

Symptoms	%	Alternate-personality characteristics	%
Markedly different moods	94	Amnestic personalities	100
Exhibiting an alter	84	Personalities with proper names (e.g., Nick, Sally)	98
Different accents	68	Angry alternate personality	80
Inability to remember angry outbursts	58	Depressed alternate personality	74
Inner conversations	58	Personalities of different ages	66
Different handwriting	34	Suicidal alternate personality	62
Different dress or makeup	32	Protector alternate personality	30
Unfamiliar people know them well	18	Self-abusive alternate personality	30
Amnesia for a previously learned subject	14	Opposite-sexed alternate personality	26
Discovery of unfamiliar possessions	14	Personality with non-proper names (e.g., "observer," "teacher")	24
Different handedness	14	Unnamed alternate personality	18

Source. Adapted from Coons PM, Bowman ES, Milstein V: "Multiple Personality Disorder. A Clinical Investigation of 50 Cases." *Journal of Nervous and Mental Diseases* 176(9):519–527, 1988.

particularly common. Borderline personality disorder, found in up to 70% of DID patients, is diagnosed on the basis of mood instability, identity disturbance, deliberate self-harm, and other characteristic symptoms. Many DID patients report psychotic symptoms such as auditory hallucinations ("voices"), and many will have a previous diagnosis of schizophrenia, schizoaffective disorder, or psychotic mood disorder.

There is no standard treatment for DID, but many clinicians recommend long-term individual psychotherapy to help patients integrate their many alters. Cognitive-behavioral therapy also has been used to help patients achieve reintegration. Although the core features of DID do not respond to medication, patients often have co-occurring mood and anxiety disorders that can benefit from drug treatment.

Dissociative Amnesia

Dissociative amnesia is defined as the inability to recall important autobiographical information that is considered too extensive to be explained by ordinary forgetfulness. With dissociative amnesia, the person typically is confused and perplexed and might not recall significant personal information or even his or her own name. The amnesia can develop suddenly and last minutes to days or longer.

The prevalence of dissociative amnesia has been estimated to be approximately 1%–3% in the general population. It affects more women than men and has been reported to occur after severe physical or psychosocial stressors (e.g., natural disasters, war).

Dissociative fugue is a subtype of dissociative amnesia that is characterized by the inability to recall one's past and assuming a new identity, which may be partial or complete. The fugue usually involves sudden, unexpected travel away from home or one's workplace, is not due to DID, and is not induced by a substance or a general medical condition (e.g., temporal lobe epilepsy). Fugue states are reported to result from psychologically stressful situations, such as natural disasters or war.

The differential diagnosis of dissociative amnesia includes many medical and neurological conditions that can cause memory impairment (e.g., a brain tumor, closed head trauma, dementia) as well as the effects of a substance (e.g., alcohol-related blackouts). A medical workup should include a physical examination, mental status examination, toxicological studies, an electroencephalogram, and other tests when indicated (e.g., magnetic resonance imaging brain scan).

As a general rule, onset and termination of amnestic states due to a medical condition or a substance are unlikely to be associated with psychological stress. Memory impairment caused by a brain injury is likely to be more severe for recent rather than for remote events and to resolve slowly if at all; in these cases, memory only rarely recovers fully. Disturbances in attention, orientation, and affect are characteristic of many brain disorders (e.g., tumors, strokes, Alzheimer's disease) but are unlikely in dissociative amnesia. Memory loss from alcohol intoxication (i.e., blackouts) is characterized by impaired short-term recall and evidence of heavy substance abuse. *Malingering* involves reporting amnesia for behaviors that are alleged to be out of character when obvious reasons exist for secondary gain (e.g., claiming amnesia about a crime).

There is no established treatment for dissociative amnesia or fugue, and recovery tends to occur spontaneously. In fugue states, recovery of past memories and resumption of the individual's former identity could occur abruptly (i.e., over several hours) but can take much longer. When memories return, help patients understand the reason for their memory loss and reinforce healthy coping mechanisms.

Depersonalization/Derealization Disorder

Depersonalization/derealization disorder is characterized by feeling detached from oneself or one's surroundings, as though one were an outside observer; some patients experience a dreamlike state. Depersonalization could be accompanied by *derealization*, a sense of detachment, unreality, and altered relation to the outside world. In DSM-IV, depersonalization and derealization were separate disorders, but in DSM-5 the two syndromes have been merged. The prevalence of depersonalization/derealization disorder is approximately 2% in the general population. It is equally common among men and women. The disorder typically begins during adolescence or early adulthood and rarely after age 40. The duration of depersonalization/derealization episodes is variable, but episodes can last hours, days, or even weeks. Reoccurrences can follow psychologically stressful situations, such as the loss of an important relationship.

Mental disorders in which depersonalization/derealization symptoms sometimes occur, such as schizophrenia, major depressive disorder, phobias, panic disorder, obsessive-compulsive disorder, PTSD, and drug abuse, must be ruled out. Medical conditions (e.g., partial complex seizures, migraine), sleep deprivation, and drug-induced states need to be ruled out as well.

There are no standard treatments, although benzodiazepines could help reduce the accompanying anxiety (e.g., diazepam, 5 mg three times daily). Selective serotonin reuptake inhibitors and clomipramine have been reported to relieve symptoms of depersonalization. Patients have reported benefit with hypnosis or cognitive-behavioral therapy to help control their episodes of depersonalization/derealization.

Clinical Points for Dissociative Disorders

- Rule out medical conditions (e.g., tumors, temporal lobe epilepsy) as a cause of the amnesia, dissociation, or depersonalization/derealization.

- Be patient and supportive. In most cases of amnesia, memory returns rapidly and completely.

- Patients with DID are especially challenging, and therapy may be long-term. The clinician might want to consider referring the patient to a therapist with experience treating the disorder.

  - It may be best to help the patient gradually learn about the number and nature of his or her alters.

  - A goal with these patients should be to help them function better and to bring about better communication among the alters.

- Medications have no proven benefit for treating dissociative disorders, although antidepressants might help some patients with depersonalization/derealization disorder.

  - Benzodiazepines may help reduce the anxiety that often accompanies depersonalization.

Further Reading

Boysen GA, VanBergen A: A review of published research on adult dissociative identity disorder: 2000-2010. J Nerv Ment Dis 201(1):5–11, 2013

Brand BL, Classen CC, McNary SW, Zaveri P: A review of dissociative disorders treatment studies. J Nerv Ment Dis 197(9):646–654, 2009

Butler LD: Normative dissociation. Psychiatr Clin North Am 29(1):45–62, 2006

Coons PM, Bowman ES, Milstein V: Multiple personality disorder. A clinical investigation of 50 cases. J Nerv Ment Dis 176(9):519–527, 1988

Foote B, Smolin Y, Kaplan M, et al: Prevalence of dissociative disorders in psychiatric outpatients. Am J Psychiatry 163(4):623–629, 2006

Lauer J, Black DW, Keen P: Multiple personality disorder and borderline personality disorder. Distinct entities or variations on a common theme? Ann Clin Psychiatry 5(2):129–134, 1993

Lowenstein RJ: Psychopharmacologic treatments of dissociative identity disorder. Psychiatr Ann 35:666–673, 2005

Simeon D, Gross S, Guralnik O, et al: Feeling unreal: 30 cases of DSM-III-R depersonalization disorder. Am J Psychiatry 154(8):1107–1113, 1997

Spiegel D, Loewenstein RJ, Lewis-Fernández R, et al: Dissociative disorders in DSM-5. Depress Anxiety 28(9):824–852, 2011

Vermetten E, Schmahl C, Lindner S, et al: Hippocampal and amygdalar volumes in dissociative identity disorder. Am J Psychiatry 163(4):630–636, 2006

Chapter 10

Somatic Symptom and Related Disorders

Somatic symptom disorders are characterized by physical symptoms that defy medical investigation. They cause significant distress to individuals and can cause serious functional impairment. In DSM-5, the somatic symptom disorders have been reconceptualized. A new diagnosis—*somatic symptom disorder*—merges DSM-IV's somatization disorder, hypochondriasis, pain disorder, and undifferentiated somatoform disorder. These four diagnoses were used rarely and created confusion for clinicians and patients.

DSM-5 somatic symptom and related disorders are listed in Table 10–1.

Somatic Symptom Disorders

Somatic Symptom Disorder

Somatic symptom disorder is characterized by the presence of one or more somatic symptoms that are distressing and/or result in significant disruption in daily life. To qualify for the diagnosis, the concerns have to have been present for at least 6 months, but not necessarily with any one symptom continuously. *Symptom migration*, in which an individual previously preoccupied with a particular symptom will focus on a new symptom, is common. When the symptom predominantly involves pain, it can be specified by the clinician ("with predominant pain"). The DSM-5 criteria for somatic symptom disorder are shown in Box 10–1.

Box 10–1. DSM-5 Criteria for Somatic Symptom Disorder

A. One or more somatic symptoms that are distressing or result in significant disruption of daily life.
B. Excessive thoughts, feelings, or behaviors related to the somatic symptoms or associated health concerns as manifested by at least one of the following:

  1. Disproportionate and persistent thoughts about the seriousness of one's symptoms.
  2. Persistently high level of anxiety about health or symptoms.
  3. Excessive time and energy devoted to these symptoms or health concerns.

C. Although any one somatic symptom may not be continuously present, the state of being symptomatic is persistent (typically more than 6 months).

TABLE 10–1. DSM-5 somatic symptom and related disorders

Somatic symptom disorder

Illness anxiety disorder

Conversion disorder (functional neurological symptom disorder)

Psychological factors affecting other medical conditions

Factitious disorder (imposed on self and imposed on another)

For individuals with somatic symptom disorders, health concerns typically trump all others, including work and family obligations. They might see their medical complaints as unduly threatening and fear the potential seriousness of them (i.e., Could this mole be a melanoma? Is this swelling a tumor?). Complaints can involve multiple organ systems and can present in dramatic fashion. As an illustration, the many symptoms reported by one of our somatic symptom disorder patients are shown in Table 10–2.

Individuals with somatic symptom disorder tend to invest substantial time and energy in their symptoms and health concerns. Quality of life often is significantly impaired, particularly when the disorder leads to a high level of

TABLE 10–2. Medical symptoms reported by a patient with a somatic symptom disorder

Organ system	Complaint
Neuropsychiatric	"The two hemispheres of my brain aren't working properly." "I couldn't name familiar objects around the house when asked." "I was hospitalized with tingling and numbness all over, and the doctors didn't know why."
Cardiopulmonary	"I had extreme dizziness after climbing stairs." "It hurts to breathe." "My heart was racing and pounding and thumping. . . . I thought I was going to die."
Gastrointestinal	"For 10 years I was treated for nervous stomach, spastic colon, and gallbladder, and nothing the doctor did seemed to help." "I got a violent cramp after eating an apple and felt terrible the next day." "The gas was awful—I thought I was going to explode."
Genitourinary	"I'm not interested in sex, but I pretend to be to satisfy my husband's needs." "I've had red patches on my labia, and I was told to use boric acid." "I had difficulty with bladder control and was examined for a tipped bladder, but nothing was found." "I had nerves cut going into my uterus because of severe cramps."
Musculoskeletal	"I have learned to live with weakness and tiredness all the time." "I thought I pulled a back muscle, but my chiropractor says it's a disc problem."
Sensory	"My vision is blurry. It's like seeing through a fog, but the doctor said that glasses wouldn't help." "I suddenly lost my hearing. It came back, but now I have whistling noises, like an echo."
Metabolic/ endocrine	"I began teaching half days because I couldn't tolerate the cold." "I was losing hair faster than my husband."

medical care. For some patients, this means frequent clinic visits, "doctor shopping," emergency department visits, hospital stays, and unnecessary medical procedures. Their preoccupation with medical symptoms typically begins early in life and can last years or even decades.

The prevalence of somatic symptom disorder is 5%–7% in the general population but higher in primary care. Women tend to report more somatic symptoms; therefore, it is more prevalent among women than among men. Onset of the disorder typically is in the 20s, although excessive health worries can begin even in geriatric patients. Low education and low income are risk factors for the disorder. Many women with somatic symptom disorder report histories of childhood sexual abuse.

The differential diagnosis of somatic symptom disorder includes panic disorder, major depression, and schizophrenia. Patients with panic disorder typically report multiple autonomic symptoms (e.g., palpitations, shortness of breath), but they occur almost exclusively during panic attacks. Patients with major depression often report multiple physical complaints, but these are overshadowed by the dysphoria and vegetative symptoms of depression (e.g., appetite loss, lack of energy, insomnia). Patients with schizophrenia sometimes have physical complaints, but the complaints often are bizarre or delusional.

Illness Anxiety Disorder

Illness anxiety disorder is new in DSM-5 and is for patients preoccupied with the possibility of having or acquiring a serious illness. The DSM-5 criteria for illness anxiety disorder are shown in Box 10–2. In DSM-IV, many of these patients would have been diagnosed with hypochondriasis. The person might amplify normal physiological sensations and misinterpret them as signs of disease, yet the distress comes mainly from his or her anxiety regarding the meaning, significance, or cause of the symptoms, and not the symptoms themselves.

Box 10–2.   DSM-5 Criteria for Illness Anxiety Disorder

A. Preoccupation with having or acquiring a serious illness.
B. Somatic symptoms are not present or, if present, are only mild in intensity. If another medical condition is present or there is a high risk for developing a medical condition (e.g., strong

family history is present), the preoccupation is clearly excessive or disproportionate.

C. There is a high level of anxiety about health, and the individual is easily alarmed about personal health status.

D. The individual performs excessive health-related behaviors (e.g., repeatedly checks his or her body for signs of illness) or exhibits maladaptive avoidance (e.g., avoids doctor appointments and hospitals).

E. Illness preoccupation has been present for at least 6 months, but the specific illness that is feared may change over that period of time.

F. The illness-related preoccupation is not better explained by another mental disorder, such as somatic symptom disorder, panic disorder, generalized anxiety disorder, body dysmorphic disorder, obsessive-compulsive disorder, or delusional disorder, somatic type.

If a physical sign or symptom is present, it often is a normal physiological sensation, a benign and self-limited dysfunction, or a bodily discomfort not generally considered indicative of disease. If a diagnosable medical condition is present, the person's anxiety and preoccupation are disproportionate to its severity. Individuals with this condition are easily alarmed about ill health and often cannot be reassured by negative medical tests or a benign course. Their preoccupation with the idea of having a serious illness directs attention away from other activities and undermines relationships.

The prevalence of illness anxiety disorder is estimated to be 1%–10% of the general population and is equally common in men and women. The disorder generally is thought to be chronic or relapsing and to have onset in early and middle adulthood.

Physicians find patients with illness anxiety disorder to be frustrating and difficult. Patients, on the other hand, feel ignored or rejected by physicians or are made to feel ashamed by those who tell them that their complaints are not legitimate. People with this condition could "doctor-shop" and receive unnecessary evaluations, tests, or surgeries. They also are at risk for alcohol or drug addiction.

Other causes of health preoccupations need to be ruled out, as well as medical conditions. Health complaints can be common among persons with mood or anxiety disorders. Individuals with obsessive-compulsive disorder will have other symptoms (e.g., hand-washing rituals). Although individuals with panic disorder might have concerns about having a heart attack, such concerns occur in the context of a panic attack.

Conversion Disorder
(Functional Neurological Symptom Disorder)

In DSM-5, conversion disorder (functional neurological symptom disorder) is defined by the presence of one or more symptoms of altered voluntary motor or sensory function that suggest a neurological or medical condition. The DSM-5 criteria for conversion disorder are shown in Box 10–3. Notably, patients whose primary complaint is limited to pain receive a diagnosis of *somatic symptom disorder*. In DSM-III and DSM-IV, psychological factors were linked with development and expression of the symptoms. The authors of DSM-5 concluded that this requirement was too difficult to prove and set the bar too high for the diagnosis, and therefore it was dropped.

Box 10–3.   DSM-5 Criteria for Conversion Disorder (Functional Neurological Symptom Disorder)

A. One or more symptoms of altered voluntary motor or sensory function.
B. Clinical findings provide evidence of incompatibility between the symptom and recognized neurological or medical conditions.
C. The symptom or deficit is not better explained by another medical or mental disorder.
D. The symptom or deficit causes clinically significant distress or impairment in social, occupational, or other important areas of functioning or warrants medical evaluation.

Symptoms of conversion disorder are common in hospital and clinic settings. For example, an estimated 20%–25% of patients admitted to neurology wards have conversion symptoms. Conversion symptoms are more frequent in women, among rural residents, and among persons with lower levels of education and income. Onset tends to be in late childhood or early adulthood. Typical symptoms include paralysis, abnormal movements, inability to speak (aphonia), blindness, and deafness. Non-epileptic seizures (often referred to as *pseudoseizures*) also are common and could occur in patients with true convulsive disorders. (These are spells that resemble true seizures but are not accompanied by abnormal brain waves.)

The cause of conversion disorder is not well understood, but most individuals who receive the diagnosis have another mental disorder, such as a mood disorder, a somatic symptom disorder, or a psychotic disorder. Conversion disorder often is associated with dissociative symptoms, such as depersonalization, derealization, and dissociative amnesia, particularly at symptom onset or during attacks.

Although most conversion symptoms are temporary, favorable outcome generally is associated with acute onset, a precipitating stressor, good premorbid adjustment, and the absence of medical or neurological comorbidity. When conversion symptoms occur in the context of another mental disorder such as major depression, outcome usually reflects the course of the primary disorder.

Clinical Management of Somatic Symptom Disorders

There are several important principles that guide treatment of somatic symptom disorders. First, the physician should follow the Hippocratic Oath and "do no harm." Because symptoms often are embellished or misidentified, physicians tend to overreact and pursue unnecessary diagnostic evaluations, surgical procedures, or medications that have little relevance to the underlying condition.

Regularly scheduled clinic visits could reduce unnecessary use of health care resources by these patients. Listen attentively and convey genuine concern but refrain from focusing on the symptoms, thereby communicating that somatic complaints are not the most important or interesting feature of the patient. Your goal becomes one of helping the patient cope with symptoms and enable him or her to function at the highest possible level.

Prescribe psychotropic medications and analgesics with caution. These medications are rarely indicated unless prescribed for a co-occurring mental disorder known to respond to the agent (e.g., antidepressants for major depression). Avoid benzodiazepines because of their abuse potential.

These simple measures have been shown to lower health care costs in patients with DSM-IV's somatization disorder and appear to reduce the likelihood of doctor-shopping and undergoing costly and unnecessary tests and procedures.

A patient with illness anxiety disorder might further benefit from cognitive-behavioral therapy that involves education about illness attitudes and selective perception of symptoms. Selective serotonin reuptake inhibitors may be effective in treating illness anxiety disorder and DSM-IV hypochondriasis.

The treatment of conversion disorder is not well established, but the goal is to reduce symptoms. Reassurance and gentle suggestion (e.g., the idea that gradual improvement is expected) are appropriate, along with efforts to resolve stressful situations that might accompany the symptoms. The rate of spontaneous remission for acute conversion symptoms is high, so that even without any specific intervention, most patients will improve.

Clinical Points for
Somatic Symptom Disorders

- Validate the patient's suffering and acknowledge his or her symptoms.

- Establish an empathic relationship to reduce the patient's tendency to doctor-shop.

  - The primary physician preferably should become the patient's only physician.

- Keep in mind that patients benefit from brief, scheduled visits.

  - As the patient improves, the time between visits can be extended.

- Remember that the physician's goal is not to remove symptoms but to improve function and quality of life.

- Minimize the use of psychotropic drugs.

  - No specific medication has proven value in somatic symptom disorder.

  - Illness anxiety disorder might respond to selective serotonin reuptake inhibitors.

  - Avoid psychotropic drugs with abuse potential (e.g., benzodiazepines, opioids).

- Minimize medical evaluations to reduce expense and iatrogenic complications.

  - Conservative management has been shown to reduce health care costs.

Psychological Factors Affecting Other Medical Conditions

The essential feature of psychological factors affecting other medical conditions is the presence of one or more clinically significant psychological or behavioral factors that adversely affect a medical condition by increasing the risk for suffering, death, or disability. These factors can adversely affect the medical condition by influencing its course or treatment, by adding a health risk factor, or by exacerbating the physiology related to the medical condition. Psychological or behavioral factors include psychological distress, patterns of interpersonal interaction, coping styles, and maladaptive help behaviors such as denying symptoms or poor adherence to medical recommendations. Common examples are a patient with anxiety that exacerbates his or her asthma, a patient who denies the need for treatment of acute chest pain, or a person with diabetes who manipulates his or her insulin in order to lose weight.

Factitious Disorder

Factitious disorder is characterized by intentional producing or feigning of physical or psychological signs or symptoms. Patients with factitious disorder have no obvious external incentives for the behavior, such as economic gain. Instead, these individuals are thought to be motivated by an unconscious desire to inhabit the sick role. Some factitious disorder patients make hospitalization a way of life. The term *Munchausen syndrome* has been used to describe patients who move from hospital to hospital simulating various illnesses.

The prevalence of factitious disorder is unknown but has been estimated to occur in about 1% of hospitalized patients. In rare cases, factitious disorder can be imposed on another person. For example, a parent induces (or simulates) illness in his or her child so that the child is hospitalized repeatedly.

Most cases of factitious disorder involve the simulation of physical illness. Patients typically use one of three strategies to feign illness:

- Reporting symptoms suggesting an illness without having the symptoms

- Producing false evidence of an illness (e.g., a factitious fever produced by applying friction to a thermometer)
- Producing symptoms of illness (e.g., by injecting feces to produce infection or by taking warfarin to induce a bleeding disorder)

Factitious disorder often begins in early adulthood and can become chronic. Many patients with factitious disorders have worked in health care occupations. Diagnostic clues include a lengthy and involved medical history that does not correspond to the patient's apparent health and vigor, a clinical presentation that too closely resembles textbook descriptions, a sophisticated medical vocabulary, demands for specific medications or treatments, and a history of excessive surgeries.

Treatment of factitious disorder is difficult. The first task is to make the diagnosis so that additional and potentially harmful medical procedures can be avoided. Because many of these patients are hospitalized on medical and surgical wards, a consulting psychiatrist can help make the diagnosis and educate the treatment team about factitious disorders. The patient should be confronted in a nonthreatening manner by the attending physician and the consulting psychiatrist.

Malingering

In DSM-5, malingering is included in the category "Other Conditions That May Be a Focus of Clinical Attention" that are not considered attributable to a mental disorder (i.e., "Z code" diagnoses). Malingering is the intentional production of false or grossly exaggerated physical or psychological symptoms motivated by external incentives, such as avoiding military duty or work, obtaining financial compensation, evading criminal prosecution, obtaining drugs, or securing better living conditions. Most malingerers are men with obvious reasons to feign illness (e.g., homelessness).

Clinicians should suspect malingering when there is a marked discrepancy between the person's claimed disability and objective findings; lack of cooperation during the diagnostic evaluation and noncompliance with the treatment regimen; and the presence of an antisocial personality disorder. Symptoms reported by malingering patients often are vague, subjective, and unverifiable.

As with factitious disorder patients, many experts believe that malingerers should be confronted with evidence that confirms the diagnosis. Others feel that confrontation simply disrupts the doctor–patient relationship and makes the patient even more alert to possible future detection. Clinicians who take the second position feel that the best approach is to treat the patient as though the symptoms were real. The symptoms can then be abandoned in response to treatment without the patient losing face.

Further Reading

Allen LA, Escobar JI, Lehrer PM, et al: Psychosocial treatments for multiple unexplained physical symptoms: a review of the literature. Psychosom Med 64(6):939–950, 2002

Barsky AJ, Fama JM, Bailey ED, Ahern DK: A prospective 4- to 5-year study of DSM-III-R hypochondriasis. Arch Gen Psychiatry 55(8):737–744, 1998

de Waal MWM, Arnold IA, Eekhof JAH, van Hemert AM: Somatoform disorders in general practice: prevalence, functional impairment and comorbidity with anxiety and depressive disorders. Br J Psychiatry 184:470–476, 2004

Dimsdale JE, Xin Y, Kleinman A, et al (eds): Somatic Presentations of Mental Disorders: Refining the Research Agenda for DSM-5. Arlington, VA, American Psychiatric Association, 2009

Fallon BA, Ahern DK, Pavlicova M, et al: A randomized controlled trial of medication and cognitive-behavioral therapy for hypochondriasis. Am J Psychiatry 174(8):756–764, 2017

Henningsen P, Jakobsen T, Schiltenwolf M, Weiss MG: Somatization revisited: diagnosis and perceived causes of common mental disorders. J Nerv Ment Dis 193(2):85–92, 2005

Krem MM: Motor conversion disorders reviewed from a neuropsychiatric perspective. J Clin Psychiatry 65(6):783–790, 2004

Noyes R, Reich J, Clancy J, O'Gorman TW: Reduction in hypochondriasis with treatment of panic disorder. Br J Psychiatry 149:631–635, 1986

Noyes R Jr, Holt CS, Kathol RG: Somatization: diagnosis and management. Arch Fam Med 4(9):790–795, 1995

Turner M: Malingering. Br J Psychiatry 171:409–411, 1997

Chapter 11

Feeding and Eating Disorders

Feeding and eating disorders involve disturbed eating behaviors that can span the entire age range. This chapter combines feeding disorders usually diagnosed in childhood with the classic eating disorders because of their shared phenomenology and pathophysiology. Binge-eating disorder has been added to DSM-5 on the basis of accumulating research over the past decade. Table 11–1 lists the DSM-5 feeding and eating disorders.

Feeding Disorders

Pica

Pica is diagnosed when a person consumes nonnutritive, nonfood substances (e.g., dirt) on a persistent basis for a period of at least 1 month. Pica has been observed in pregnant women, in persons with intellectual disability, and in those with specific medical disorders (e.g., iron deficiency). Children up to age 24 months frequently mouth—or even eat—nonnutritive items; this is considered developmentally normal. Therefore, a minimum age of 2 years is suggested for a pica diagnosis. There is no specific treatment for pica. Behavioral therapy that emphasizes and rewards appropriate eating behavior, or that negatively reinforces nonnutritive food consumption, has been recommended.

Rumination Disorder

With rumination disorder a person repeatedly regurgitates swallowed or partially digested food, which is then either re-chewed, re-swallowed, or expelled. Young children are most likely to re-chew regurgitated food. There is no retching, nausea, heartburn, odors, or abdominal pains associated with the regurgitation, as is typical with vomiting. The disorder is more

TABLE 11–1. DSM-5 feeding and eating disorders

Pica

Rumination disorder

Avoidant/restrictive food intake disorder

Anorexia nervosa

Bulimia nervosa

Binge-eating disorder

common among infants, young children, and individuals with developmental disabilities. The regurgitation often is effortless and unforced. As with pica, there are no specific treatments for the condition, but behavioral therapy that rewards nonrumination with parental attention has been recommended.

Avoidant/Restrictive Food Intake Disorder

Avoidant/restrictive food intake disorder is characterized by a disturbance of eating or feeding behavior that takes the form of avoiding or restricting food intake. There are three main subtypes of affected individuals:

- Individuals who do not eat enough or show little interest in feeding or eating
- Individuals who accept only a limited diet in relation to sensory features
- Individuals whose food refusal is related to aversive experience

Avoidance or restriction associated with insufficient intake or lack of interest in food usually develops in infancy or early childhood, although it can begin in adolescence; onset in adulthood is rare. The diagnosis does not apply to children who are picky eaters, older persons with reduced food intake, or pregnant women who do not eat certain foods because of altered sensory sensitivities. Avoidant/restrictive food intake disorder is equally common among males and females in infancy and childhood.

Although avoidant/restrictive food intake disorder could resemble anorexia nervosa because of resulting weight loss, the disorder is not associated with fear of gaining weight or distorted perceptions about one's body weight or shape.

Eating Disorders

Anorexia nervosa and *bulimia nervosa*, the two major eating disorders, are each associated with disturbed eating behaviors occurring in persons who are intensely preoccupied with food, body weight, and body shape. To these, DSM-5 has added *binge-eating disorder*, which is characterized by binge eating in the absence of compensatory behaviors.

Anorexia Nervosa

Anorexia nervosa is associated with significant weight loss—defined as a "restriction of energy intake relative to requirements, leading to a significantly low body weight"—occurring in the presence of an intense fear of gaining weight or of becoming fat or persistent behavior that interferes with weight gain, and a disturbance in the perception of body shape. The clinician can specify whether the disorder is the *restricting type* (i.e., no bingeing or purging) or the *binge-eating/purging type*. The DSM-5 criteria for anorexia nervosa are shown in Box 11–1.

Box 11–1.   DSM-5 Criteria for Anorexia Nervosa

A. Restriction of energy intake relative to requirements, leading to a significantly low body weight in the context of age, sex, developmental trajectory, and physical health. *Significantly low weight* is defined as a weight that is less than minimally normal or, for children and adolescents, less than that minimally expected.

B. Intense fear of gaining weight or of becoming fat, or persistent behavior that interferes with weight gain, even though at a significantly low weight.

C. Disturbance in the way in which one's body weight or shape is experienced, undue influence of body weight or shape on self-evaluation, or persistent lack of recognition of the seriousness of the current low body weight.

Body mass index (BMI; weight in kilograms/height in meters^2) is a critical measure for assessing body weight and size. Most adults with a BMI ≥ 18.5 are not considered significantly underweight. Those with a BMI < 17 are considered significantly underweight. People with anorexia nervosa are subtyped as *mild, moderate, severe,* or *extreme* based on BMI.

The discrepancy between weight and perceived body image is key to diagnosing anorexia nervosa. Individuals with anorexia nervosa delight in their weight loss and fear gaining weight. Persons with bulimia can successfully hide their binge-eating and purging behaviors and often have normal weight. In practice, the two syndromes tend to intertwine, meaning that patients often have a mixture of symptoms.

Bulimia Nervosa

Bulimia nervosa consists of the following:

- Recurrent episodes of binge eating;
- A feeling of lack of control over eating during the binges;
- Recurrent use of inappropriate compensatory behaviors to prevent weight gain, such as vomiting, use of laxatives or diuretics, strict dieting or fasting, or vigorous exercise;
- An average of at least one binge episode weekly for 3 months; and
- Persistent overconcern with body shape and weight.

Binge-Eating Disorder

Binge-eating disorder involves the following:

- Recurrent binge eating without compensatory behaviors such as purging or excessive exercising.

The distinction between binge-eating disorder and bulimia nervosa sometimes is unclear, and the two diagnoses may represent different stages of the same underlying disorder. Compared with people with bulimia nervosa, people with binge-eating disorder generally are older, are more likely to be male, and experience onset at an older age. Nearly two-thirds of individuals with binge-eating disorder have a history of using inappropriate compensatory behaviors, suggesting a previous diagnosis of bulimia nervosa.

Epidemiology of Eating Disorders

An estimated 1% of women have anorexia nervosa, while up to 4% have bulimia nervosa. For either disorder, the frequency in men is approximately one-tenth that in women. Isolated symptoms, such as binge eating, purging (e.g., self-induced vomiting), or fasting, are far more common than the disorders themselves. Binge-eating disorder could be the most frequent eating disorder in the general population, affecting 3.5% of women and 2% of men.

Eating disorders typically have an onset during adolescence or young adulthood. Anorexia nervosa often has an earlier onset (early teens) than bulimia nervosa (late teens, early 20s). Eating disorders are found in all social strata, although they were once thought to be more common in the higher socioeconomic groups. Anorexia nervosa is uncommon in non-industrialized countries and is less frequent among African Americans. Eating disorders are overrepresented in occupations that require rigorous control of body shape (e.g., modeling, ballet dancing).

Clinical Findings

A person with anorexia nervosa develops elaborate behaviors designed to promote weight loss. They typically are preoccupied with food and food preparation, nutrition, and special diets (e.g., vegetarian), interests that belie their fear of gaining weight. Abuse of laxatives, diuretics, or stimulants in an effort to enhance weight loss is common.

Binge eating and purging tend to occur in private. Binges involve consuming large amounts of food in a short period of time. Compensatory behaviors develop as a way to counteract the binge or its perceived effects, and include self-induced vomiting (purging), laxative use, and over-exercise.

People with anorexia nervosa can develop profound weight loss. In addition to looking emaciated, they often have hypothermia, dependent edema, bradycardia, and hypotension. Some persons develop sensitivity to temperature and report feeling cold much of the time. Near-chronic constipation leads many patients to become dependent on laxatives. Hormonal abnormalities, including elevated growth hormone levels, increased plasma cortisol, and reduced gonadotropin levels, can develop. Thyroxin and thyroid-stimulating hormone can be normal even when triiodothyronine (T_3) is reduced. Men with anorexia nervosa generally have low levels of circulating testosterone and can show clinical signs of hypogonadism. Amenorrhea precedes the onset of observable weight loss in one-fifth of female patients, although it is not required for the diagnosis.

Bulimia can cause serious dental problems, including erosion of tooth enamel and multiple caries. Esophageal erosion or tears caused by the force of repeated vomiting can occur.

Medical complications of bulimic behavior are summarized in Table 11–2.

Course and Outcome

The long-term course of eating disorders ranges from full recovery to malignant weight loss and rapid death. About 25%–40% of eating disorder patients have a good outcome, meaning that they eat normally, do not binge or purge, and are emotionally well adjusted. In the remaining patients, the characteristic symptoms of the illness (e.g., distorted body image, abnormal eating behaviors) persist.

Diagnosis and Assessment

Diagnosis rests on the patient's history and mental status examination. Assessment should include a thorough physical examination, with special attention given to vital signs, weight, skin quality and turgor, and the cardiovascular system. The patient's weight and height should be measured so that the appropriateness of weight for height, age, and gender can be determined.

Laboratory studies can help to rule out other medical conditions, such as malabsorption syndromes, hyperthyroidism, and midline tumors in the brain. The workup should include a complete blood count, urinalysis, blood urea nitrogen, and serum electrolytes. For malnourished and severely symptomatic patients, other tests are recommended, including serum cholesterol and lipids; serum calcium, magnesium, phosphorus, and amylase; liver enzymes; and an electrocardiogram. Brain imaging with magnetic resonance or computed tomography is indicated in some patients to rule out a mass lesion. Thyroid function tests are needed when hyperthyroidism is suspected as a cause of weight loss. Bone mineral densitometry is helpful in assessing and monitoring osteoporosis; bone-density measurements are more than two standard deviations below normal in approximately one-half of women with anorexia nervosa.

Rule out other mental disorders as the cause of disturbed eating behavior, including schizophrenia, major depressive disorder, obsessive-compulsive disorder, and other eating disorders. Comorbid major depressive disorder is common among these patients, as are anxiety disorders and personality disorders.

TABLE 11–2. Medical complications of eating disorders

Physical manifestations

Amenorrhea

Sensitivity to cold

Constipation

Low blood pressure

Bradycardia

Hypothermia

Lanugo hair

Hair loss

Petechia

Carotenemic skin

Parotid gland enlargement[a]

Dental erosion, caries[a]

Pedal edema

Dry skin

Endocrine abnormalities

Increased growth hormone levels

Increased plasma cortisol and loss of diurnal variation

Reduced gonadotropin levels (LH, FSH, impaired response to LHRH)

Low T_3, high T_3RU, impaired TRH responsiveness[a]

Abnormal glucose tolerance test results

Abnormal dexamethasone suppression test results[a]

Laboratory abnormalities

Dehydration[a]

Hypokalemia[a]

Hypochloremia[a]

Alkalosis

Leukopenia

Elevated transaminases

Elevated serum cholesterol

Carotenemia

Elevated BUN[a]

Elevated amylase levels[a]

Note. BUN=blood urea nitrogen; FSH=follicle-stimulating hormone; LH= luteinizing hormone; LHRH=luteinizing hormone–releasing hormone; T_3=triiodothyronine; T_3RU=triiodothyronine reuptake; TRH=thyrotropin-releasing hormone.
[a]Seen in patients who binge and purge.

Clinical Management

With eating disorders, there are three basic treatment goals that aim to

- Restore a normal nutritional state. For patients with anorexia nervosa, this means restoring weight to within a normal range. For persons with bulimia, this means ensuring that metabolic balance is achieved.
- Modify the patients' disturbed eating behaviors. This will help the patient maintain his or her weight within a normal range and reverse (or lessen) binge eating, purging, and other abnormal eating behaviors.
- Help change the patient's erroneous beliefs about food, weight loss, and body size/shape.

Treatment generally involves behavioral modification combined with individual and group psychotherapy. The purpose of behavioral therapy is to restore normal eating behavior. This is accomplished by setting goals for both eating and weight gain and targeting specific abnormal behaviors for correction (e.g., purging behaviors).

Some patients will need to be hospitalized to fully address the following:

- Severe starvation and weight loss, hypotension or hypothermia, and electrolyte imbalance.
- Suicidal ideation or psychosis.
- Failure of outpatient treatment, as indicated by the inability to gain weight or reverse severe binge/purge cycles.

In the hospital, the patient should be weighed regularly and daily fluid intake and output recorded. Patients should be observed for at least 2 hours after meals to prevent vomiting, even if attendants must accompany them to the bathroom. Patients typically are started on a diet that provides 500 calories more than the amount required to maintain their present weight; caloric intake is then gradually increased. Those who are significantly underweight or are having trouble gaining weight might need tube feedings.

An electrocardiogram is essential for assessing palpitations or for evaluating changes consistent with hypokalemia. Prolongation of the QT interval should lead to immediate medical intervention because it may increase the risk of ventricular tachycardia and sudden death and is a contraindication to tricyclic antidepressants. Stool softeners or bulk laxatives can help alleviate the severe constipation associated with long-term use of stimulant laxatives or their withdrawal. Administer supplemental calcium (1,000–1,500 mg/day) and a multivitamin to ensure that vitamin D intake is adequate (400 IU/day).

The selective serotonin reuptake inhibitor (SSRI) fluoxetine (60 mg/day) is FDA-approved for treating bulimia nervosa. Other SSRIs are routinely prescribed and could be as effective. Tricyclic antidepressants and monoamine oxidase inhibitors probably are effective in reducing binge and purge cycles, but they are not considered first-line agents. Bupropion is contraindicated because it can lower seizure threshold in eating disorder patients who have electrolyte disturbances. Lisdexamfetamine (Vyvanse) is FDA-approved to treat binge-eating disorder.

There are no medications FDA-approved for treating anorexia nervosa. Second-generation antipsychotics have been used in patients with anorexia nervosa and could promote weight gain and reduce cognitive distortions. Other medications are indicated when the eating disorder is accompanied by comorbid psychosis, major depressive disorder, bipolar disorder, or an anxiety disorder (e.g., an antidepressant for major depressive disorder).

Individual psychotherapy should focus on educating the patient about the eating disorder, helping the patient understand her or his symptoms, and explaining the need for treatment. Later, approaches that aim to promote insight can be used to help the patient resolve problems and conflicts that may have contributed to or reinforced the abnormal eating behavior. Family therapy often is helpful, especially if the patient is living at home. Couples therapy can be helpful to patients in a committed relationship.

Cognitive-behavioral therapy and interpersonal psychotherapy have been shown to be effective in patients with bulimia nervosa. Cognitive-behavioral therapy helps to correct inappropriate thoughts and beliefs that patients with bulimia nervosa have about themselves and their disorder. With interpersonal psychotherapy, interpersonal conflicts thought to precede or contribute to the person's disturbed eating behavior are addressed.

Clinical Points for Feeding and Eating Disorders

- Encourage an empathic relationship. This could be hard to achieve because patients with anorexia nervosa can be oppositional and might not be sufficiently motivated to make the needed changes. Some will lack insight and refuse treatment.

- Assess the patient carefully for psychiatric comorbidity.

  - The presence of psychiatric comorbidity complicates treatment and must be addressed. Patients with an eating disorder are highly likely to have comorbid major depressive disorder, anxiety disorders, substance use disorder, or a personality disorder.

  - The presence of a personality disorder, particularly from Cluster B (e.g., borderline personality disorder), is common among patients with bulimia and is associated with poor treatment response.

- Set a firm behavioral contract with patients and have them sign it.

  - Develop reasonable targets for behavioral modification.

  - Set goals and avoid changes if possible.

- Medication has limited value for treating anorexia nervosa.

- Medication is an important treatment adjunct in patients with bulimic behaviors.

  - SSRIs are the drugs of first choice; fluoxetine (60 mg/day) is the best researched, but others are likely to be effective as well (e.g., sertraline, 50–200 mg/day; paroxetine, 20–60 mg/day; escitalopram, 10–20 mg/day).

  - Tricyclic antidepressants and monoamine oxidase inhibitors are effective but are considered second-line choices because of their potential adverse effects and dangerousness in overdose.

  - Lisdexamfetamine is FDA-approved to treat binge-eating disorder.

  - Bupropion should be avoided because of its tendency to lower seizure threshold.

- Family therapy can be especially helpful with patients who live at home or whose behavior has created problems within the family.

- Couples therapy will be beneficial for those whose eating disorder has disrupted their marriage.

Further Reading

American Psychiatric Association: Practice guideline for eating disorders, third edition. Am J Psychiatry 163 (7, suppl):4–54, 2006

Bissada H, Tasca GA, Barber AM, Bradwejn J: Olanzapine in the treatment of low body weight and obsessive thinking in women with anorexia nervosa: a randomized, double-blind, placebo-controlled trial. Am J Psychiatry 165(10):1281–1288, 2008

Collier DA, Treasure JL: The aetiology of eating disorders. Br J Psychiatry 185:363–365, 2004

Garber AK, Michihata N, Hetnal K, et al: A prospective examination of weight gain in hospitalized adolescents with anorexia nervosa on a recommended refeeding protocol. J Adolesc Health 50(1):24–29, 2012

Grilo CM, Masheb RM, Wilson GT: Efficacy of cognitive behavioral therapy and fluoxetine for the treatment of binge eating disorder: a randomized double-blind placebo-controlled comparison. Biol Psychiatry 57(3):301–309, 2005

Keel PK, Mitchell JE: Outcome in bulimia nervosa. Am J Psychiatry 154(3):313–321, 1997

Lilenfeld LR, Kaye WH, Greeno CG, et al: A controlled family study of anorexia nervosa and bulimia nervosa: psychiatric disorders in first-degree relatives and effects of proband comorbidity. Arch Gen Psychiatry 55(7):603–610, 1998

Mehler PS, Andersen AE (eds): Eating Disorders: A Guide to Medical Care and Complications, 2nd Edition. Baltimore, MD, Johns Hopkins University Press, 2010

Pike KM, Carter JC, Olmsted MP: Cognitive-behavioral therapy for anorexia nervosa, in The Treatment of Eating Disorders: A Clinical Handbook. Edited by Grilo CM, Mitchell JE. New York, Guilford, 2010, pp 83–107

Yager J, Powers PS (eds): Clinical Manual of Eating Disorders. Washington, DC, American Psychiatric Publishing, 2007

Chapter 12

Sleep-Wake Disorders

The DSM-5 sleep-wake disorders chapter is strongly influenced by the second edition of the *International Classification of Sleep Disorders*, 2nd Edition (ICSD-2), published by the American Academy of Sleep Medicine in 2005. Although DSM-5 does not include as many sleep disorders (Table 12–1), the diagnoses are compatible with ICSD-2 categories.

Normal Sleep and Sleep Architecture

The average healthy adult requires 7.5–8.5 hours of sleep per night, although some persons require more or less to feel sufficiently rested. Young people tend to sleep more than older adults, whose total sleep time tends to decrease. The longer a person has been awake, the more quickly he or she will fall asleep.

Sleep stages in adults are divided into rapid eye movement (REM) and non-REM (NREM) sleep. These sleep stages alternate in a cycle that lasts 70–120 minutes. Generally, three to six NREM/REM cycles occur nightly. The first REM period lasts 5–10 minutes; during the night, REM periods become longer and closer together and show progressively greater density of REM.

The normal sleep stages in adults are shown in Table 12–2.

Assessment of Sleep

Patients with sleep complaints should receive a thorough evaluation of their medical, psychiatric, and sleep history (Table 12–3). The medical history should include a careful review of illicit drug and medication use. Patients should be asked to maintain a sleep log, in which they record their bedtime, sleep latency (estimated time required to fall asleep),

TABLE 12–1. DSM-5 sleep-wake disorders

Insomnia disorder

Hypersomnolence disorder

Narcolepsy

Breathing-related sleep disorders

  Obstructive sleep apnea hypopnea

  Central sleep apnea

  Sleep-related hypoventilation

Circadian rhythm sleep-wake disorders

Parasomnias

  Non–rapid eye movement sleep arousal disorders

  Nightmare disorder

  Rapid eye movement sleep behavior disorder

Restless legs syndrome

Substance/medication-induced sleep disorder

awake time, number of awakenings, daytime naps, and use of drugs or medications. Interviewing the patient's bed partner to learn about the presence of snoring, breathing difficulties, or leg jerks can be helpful. *Polysomnography*—a procedure in which electroencephalographic, electrooculographic, and electromyographic tracings are recorded during sleep—might be appropriate for some patients. Results can help assess narcolepsy, breathing-related sleep disorders, and rapid eye movement sleep behavior disorder. The Multiple Sleep Latency Test (MSLT) is used to measure excessive sleepiness.

Insomnia Disorder

Insomnia is relatively common among the general population and is even more prevalent among psychiatric patients. For most individuals, insomnia is transient and stress-related (e.g., prompted by job loss, marital problems) and tends to self-correct. Yet in some persons, insomnia persists and becomes chronic, causing distress and impairment. In DSM-5,

TABLE 12–2. Sleep stages in adults

Stage 0	A period of wakefulness with eyes closed that occurs just before sleep onset. Electroencephalographic (EEG) recording mainly shows sinusoidal alpha waves over the occiput. Muscle tone is increased. Alpha activity decreases as drowsiness increases.
Stage 1	A period known as the sleep-onset stage because it provides a transition from wakefulness to sleep. Alpha activity diminishes to less than 50% of the EEG recording. Stage 1 accounts for about 5% of the total sleep period.
Stage 2	A stage dominated by theta activity and appearance of sleep spindles and K complexes. *Sleep spindles* are brief bursts of rhythmic waves. *K complexes* are sharp, negative, high-voltage EEG waves, followed by slower, positive activity. Stage 2 usually accounts for 45%–55% of the total sleep time.
Stage 3	Slow-wave or deep sleep characterized by high-voltage delta wave activity. Muscle tone is increased, but eye movements are absent. This stage constitutes 15%–20% of the total sleep time.
REM sleep	A period characterized by an EEG recording similar to that seen in Stage 1, along with a burst of rapid conjugate eye movements and reduced muscle tone. REM periods occur in phasic bursts and are accompanied by respiratory and cardiac rate fluctuations and penile/clitoral engorgement. This stage constitutes 20%–25% of the total sleep period.

insomnia disorder is defined as difficulty initiating or maintaining sleep, or early morning awakening with an inability to return to sleep. The DSM-5 criteria for insomnia disorder are listed in Box 12–1.

Box 12–1.   DSM-5 Criteria for Insomnia Disorder

A. A predominant complaint of dissatisfaction with sleep quantity or quality, associated with one (or more) of the following symptoms:

1. Difficulty initiating sleep. (In children, this may manifest as difficulty initiating sleep without caregiver intervention.)

Sleep-Wake Disorders   **171**

2. Difficulty maintaining sleep, characterized by frequent awakenings or problems returning to sleep after awakenings. (In children, this may manifest as difficulty returning to sleep without caregiver intervention.)

3. Early-morning awakening with inability to return to sleep.

B. The sleep disturbance causes clinically significant distress or impairment in social, occupational, educational, academic, behavioral, or other important areas of functioning.

C. The sleep difficulty occurs at least 3 nights per week.

D. The sleep difficulty is present for at least 3 months.

E. The sleep difficulty occurs despite adequate opportunity for sleep.

F. The insomnia is not better explained by and does not occur exclusively during the course of another sleep-wake disorder (e.g., narcolepsy, a breathing-related sleep disorder, a circadian rhythm sleep-wake disorder, a parasomnia).

G. The insomnia is not attributable to the physiological effects of a substance (e.g., a drug of abuse, a medication).

H. Coexisting mental disorders and medical conditions do not adequately explain the predominant complaint of insomnia.

For many persons with insomnia disorder, "sleep hygiene" measures will be sufficient and lead to improved sleep quality:

- Waking up and going to bed at the same time every day, even on weekends
- Avoiding long periods of wakefulness in bed
- Not using the bed as a place to read, watch television, or work
- Leaving the bed and not returning until drowsy if sleep does not begin within a set period (e.g., 20 to 30 minutes)
- Avoiding napping
- Exercising at least three or four times a week (but not in the evening if it interferes with sleep)
- Discontinuing or reducing consumption of alcoholic beverages, beverages containing caffeine, cigarettes, and sedative-hypnotic and anxiolytic drugs

Some individuals can benefit from hypnotic medications (i.e., sleeping pills). Hypnotics should be used mainly to treat transient and short-term insomnia, in combination with appropriate sleep hygiene. Traditionally, benzodiazepines have

TABLE 12–3. Sleep history outline

Obtain data from the patient, chart, and nursing staff. Review medication history, including illicit drugs, alcohol, and use of sedative or hypnotic medication. Get information on the following sleep characteristics:

- Usual sleep pattern

- Characteristics of disturbed sleep (for insomnia, difficulty falling asleep, difficulty staying asleep, or early-morning awakenings)

- The clinical course: onset, duration, frequency, severity, and precipitating and relieving factors

- 24-hour sleep-wake cycle (corroborate with the staff and chart)

- History of sleep disturbances, including childhood sleep pattern and pattern of sleep when under stress

- Family history of sleep disorders

- Personal history of other sleep disorders

- Sleep pattern at home as described by the bed partner

- Consumption of alcoholic beverages; over-the-counter caffeine tablets; coffee, tea, cola, and chocolate; and herbals such as kava that may be stimulating

- Use of prescription and over-the-counter medications

been the first choice because of safety and efficacy. Several nonbenzodiazepine alternatives are available, such as zolpidem and eszopiclone. Benzodiazepine and nonbenzodiazepine hypnotics used to treat insomnia are listed in Table 12–4.

The antihistamines diphenhydramine (25–100 mg) and doxylamine (25–100 mg) often are used as hypnotics but are not as potent as benzodiazepines. The sedating antidepressant trazodone (50–200 mg) also seems to be effective. An alternative is a low-dosage formulation of the tricyclic antidepressant doxepin (Silenor), which is FDA-approved for treating insomnia characterized by difficulty with sleep maintenance. The pineal gland hormone melatonin, sold in health food stores, is often used to treat insomnia, but controlled studies show little benefit.

TABLE 12–4. Medications used to treat insomnia

Drug (trade name)	Onset	Half-life, hours	Dose range, mg
Benzodiazepines			
Estazolam (ProSom)	Very fast	10–24	1–2
Flurazepam (Dalmane)	Very fast	2[a]	15–30
Quazepam (Doral)	Very fast	15–35	7.5–15
Temazepam (Restoril)	Moderate	8–18	15–30
Triazolam (Halcion)	Very fast	2–3	0.125–0.5
Nonbenzodiazepines			
Eszopiclone (Lunesta)	Very fast	6	1–3
Ramelteon (Rozerem)	Very fast	1–3	8
Suvorexant (Belsomra)	Moderate	12	10–20
Zaleplon (Sonata)	Very fast	1	5–20
Zolpidem (Ambien)	Very fast	2–3	5–10

[a]The half-life of its major metabolite is 47–100 hours.

Hypersomnolence Disorder

Excessive daytime somnolence affects approximately 5% of the adult population. With hypersomnolence disorder, the excessive sleepiness occurs at least three times a week for at least 3 months, as evidenced by the following:

- The individual experiences prolonged sleep episodes, daytime sleep episodes, or difficulty being fully awake after abrupt awakening
- The excessive sleepiness causes significant impairment or distress.
- The excessive sleepiness is not accounted for by another sleep disorder, a medical condition or mental disorder, or the effects of a substance.

Hypersomnolence disorder usually involves prolonged nocturnal sleep and continuous daytime drowsiness. Nearly one-half of patients report *sleep drunkenness* (i.e., excessive grogginess) on awakening, which may last several hours. Patients also might take one or two naps daily, which can each last more than an hour.

Polysomnographic studies have shown diminished delta sleep, increased number of awakenings, and reduced REM latency in patients with primary hypersomnia. The MSLT can be used to document the short sleep latency.

Treatment involves a combination of sleep hygiene measures, stimulants, and naps for some patients. Stimulants can help maintain wakefulness. Dextroamphetamine and methylphenidate have relatively short half-lives and are taken in multiple divided doses. Modafinil, which is used to treat narcolepsy, can relieve hypersomnolence disorder.

Narcolepsy

Narcolepsy is characterized by recurrent episodes of an irrepressible need to sleep. These sleep attacks occur with one or more of the following:

- Episodes of cataplexy
- Cerebrospinal fluid hypocretin deficiency
- Nocturnal polysomnography showing a REM latency of ≤15 minutes or MSLT showing a mean sleep latency of ≤8 minutes

The DSM-5 criteria for narcolepsy are shown in Box 12–2.

Box 12–2. DSM-5 Criteria for Narcolepsy

A. Recurrent periods of an irrepressible need to sleep, lapsing into sleep, or napping occurring within the same day. These must have been occurring at least three times per week over the past 3 months.

B. The presence of at least one of the following:

   1. Episodes of cataplexy, defined as either (a) or (b), occurring at least a few times per month:

      a. In individuals with long-standing disease, brief (seconds to minutes) episodes of sudden bilateral loss of muscle tone with maintained consciousness that are precipitated by laughter or joking.

b. In children or in individuals within 6 months of onset, spontaneous grimaces or jaw-opening episodes with tongue thrusting or a global hypotonia, without any obvious emotional triggers.

2. Hypocretin deficiency, as measured using cerebrospinal fluid (CSF) hypocretin-1 immunoreactivity values (less than or equal to one-third of values obtained in healthy subjects tested using the same assay, or less than or equal to 110 pg/mL). Low CSF levels of hypocretin-1 must not be observed in the context of acute brain injury, inflammation, or infection.

3. Nocturnal sleep polysomnography showing rapid eye movement (REM) sleep latency less than or equal to 15 minutes, or a multiple sleep latency test showing a mean sleep latency less than or equal to 8 minutes and two or more sleep-onset REM periods.

Narcolepsy affects approximately 1 in 2,000 persons. Men and women are equally likely to develop narcolepsy. Up to one-half of patients with narcolepsy have a first-degree relative with the disorder. Mood and anxiety disorders are common in these persons. Narcolepsy is one of the few DSM-5 disorders in which a biologic mechanism has been identified and is included in the criteria. Narcolepsy nearly always is caused by the loss of hypothalamic hypocretin-producing cells, causing cerebrospinal fluid hypocretin-1 deficiency. Hypocretin is a neurotransmitter that regulates arousal, wakefulness, and appetite. Striking features include the following:

- *Sleep attacks:* These can last from seconds to 30 minutes or longer. Patients with narcolepsy can experience sleep attacks at work, during conversations, or in other situations normally considered stimulating.
- *Cataplexy:* About 70% of patients experience the sudden bilateral loss of muscle tone precipitated by laughter or joking, or by spontaneous grimaces or jaw-opening episodes without an emotional trigger.

A sleep history is helpful in making a narcolepsy diagnosis, as are descriptions provided by parents, spouses, and bed partners. Polysomnography allows the clinician to rule out other sleep disorders such as a breathing-related sleep disorder. People with narcolepsy tend to enter REM sleep quickly rather than the more typical 90–120 minutes and during daytime naps.

Treating narcolepsy involves targeting the sleep attacks and cataplexy. Stimulants are drugs for treating sleep attacks. Methylphenidate is administered in multiple divided doses starting with 5 mg; the dosage can be gradually increased to 60 mg/day; dextroamphetamine can be prescribed in similar dosages. Modafinil (200–400 mg/day) is an effective alternative FDA-approved to treat narcolepsy. Sodium oxybate is FDA-approved for treating cataplexy and has been shown to reduce the frequency of cataplexy episodes.

Breathing-Related Sleep Disorders

Disturbed breathing mechanisms can disrupt sleep and lead to potentially serious medical, social, and psychological consequences.

Obstructive Sleep Apnea Hypopnea

Obstructive sleep apnea hypopnea is the most common breathing-related sleep disorder. It can be serious because breathing repeatedly stops and starts during sleep. A pause in breathing is called an *apnea* episode, and a decrease in airflow during breathing is called a *hypopnea* episode. Most people have brief apnea episodes during sleep, but the person with obstructive sleep apnea rarely is aware of having difficulty breathing, even upon awakening.

Snoring is the most noticeable sign of obstructive sleep apnea hypopnea. The body's muscle tone ordinarily relaxes during sleep, and the soft tissue of the airway at the throat can collapse and obstruct breathing during sleep as well as produce snoring.

Obstructive sleep apnea hypopnea most commonly affects middle-age and older adults and people who are overweight. Common signs and symptoms include excessive daytime sleepiness, loud snoring, observed episodes of breathing cessation during sleep, abrupt awakenings accompanied by shortness of breath, awakening with a dry mouth or sore throat, morning headache, difficulty staying asleep, and difficult-to-control high blood pressure. Disrupted breathing impairs the ability to achieve deep, restful sleep, resulting in the person feeling sleepy during waking hours.

Serious psychological consequences include general slowing of thought processes, memory impairment, and inattention. Patients often report anxiety, dysphoric mood, or multiple physical complaints.

A thorough assessment can include a sleep laboratory evaluation with recording respiration and monitoring nocturnal oxygen desaturation. Initial treatment measures include weight loss, avoiding sedative-hypnotics, and sleep position training to encourage patients to avoid sleeping on their back. For some patients, custom-made oral appliances can help keep the airway open.

Continuous positive airway pressure (CPAP) is the most widely used treatment. Ambient air is blown into the nose through a nasal mask or cushioned cannulae. Some patients do not tolerate CPAP well, but careful follow-up can enhance compliance. Uvulopalatopharyngoplasty is a surgical alternative for patients with redundant oropharyngeal tissue. Tracheostomy is reserved for life-threatening situations in patients who do not respond to CPAP or uvulopalatopharyngoplasty.

Central Sleep Apnea

Central sleep apnea is characterized by repeated episodes of apnea and hypopnea during sleep caused by variability in respiratory effort. These occur because the brain fails to send proper signals to the muscles that control breathing.

Central sleep apnea accounts for less than 5% of sleep apnea cases. Common signs and symptoms are essentially the same as those seen in obstructive sleep apnea hypopnea. Although snoring indicates some degree of increased airflow obstruction, snoring is not uncommon in people with central sleep apnea. Central sleep apnea is associated with several conditions, including heart failure and chronic opioid use. Importantly, central and obstructive sleep apneas can coexist (i.e., *complex sleep apnea*). The clinician can specify three subtypes of central sleep apnea:

1. *Idiopathic central sleep apnea*, characterized by repeated episodes of apneas and hypopneas caused by variability in respiratory effort
2. *Cheyne-Stokes breathing*, characterized by a pattern of crescendo-decrescendo variation in tidal volume that results in central apneas and hypopneas at a frequency of at least 5 events/hour accompanied by frequent arousal

3. *Central sleep apnea comorbid with opioid use*, in which opioids suppress the respiratory drive

Treatment of central sleep apnea is similar to that for obstructive sleep apnea hypopnea. In some cases, medication
(acetazolamide, theophylline) can be prescribed to stimulate
breathing.

Sleep-Related Hypoventilation

Sleep-related hypoventilation is the result of decreased response to high carbon dioxide levels during sleep and is characterized by frequent episodes of shallow breathing lasting
more than 10 seconds during sleep. Polysomnography shows
episodes of decreased respiration associated with elevated
carbon dioxide levels. Sleep-related hypoventilation frequently is associated with lung disease or neuromuscular or
chest wall disorders.

Individuals with sleep-related hypoventilation present
with having insomnia or excessive sleepiness, feeling breath-
less when lying down (orthopnea), and having headaches
upon awakening. During sleep, episodes of shallow breathing can be observed, and obstructive sleep apnea hypopnea
or central sleep apnea can coexist. Consequences of ventilatory
insufficiency can be present, including pulmonary hypertension, cor pulmonale (right heart failure), polycythemia, and
neurocognitive dysfunction. With progression of ventilatory
insufficiency, blood gas abnormalities extend into wakefulness. Features of the medical condition causing sleep-related
hypoventilation also can be present. Idiopathic sleep-related
hypoventilation is a slowly progressive disorder of respiratory impairment. When comorbid with other disorders (e.g.,
chronic obstructive pulmonary disease, neuromuscular disorders, obesity), disease severity reflects the severity of the underlying condition.

Treatment is directed at correcting the underlying disorder. For example, bronchodilators (e.g., albuterol, salmeterol)
can be helpful when treating patients with obstructive lung
disease. Theophylline could improve diaphragm muscle con-
tractility and stimulate the respiratory center. Patients should
refrain from using respiratory depressants (e.g., alcohol, benzodiazepines). Some patients will need ventilatory assistance,
including endotracheal intubation with mechanical ventilation or noninvasive bilevel positive-pressure ventilation. En-

courage weight loss in those who are overweight, because even modest loss improves ventilation.

Circadian Rhythm Sleep-Wake Disorders

Circadian rhythm sleep-wake disorders are persistent or recurring patterns of sleep disruption that result from an altered sleep-wake schedule or that occur when the sleep-wake cycle is not correctly synchronized with a person's daily schedule. Individuals with circadian rhythm sleep-wake disorders generally are able to get enough sleep if allowed to sleep and wake at the times dictated by their body clocks; sleep usually is of normal quality.

Our body clocks (i.e., circadian cycles) are tightly linked to core body temperature, genetics, and light exposure. In constant darkness, our body clocks typically follow a 24.2-hour cycle, but they reset to a 24-hour period with morning light exposure. For this reason, people sleep best by initiating sleep when "sleep debt,"which increases linearly while one is awake, is high and the alerting system starts to wane. We wake spontaneously when sleep debt—lowered by sleep—intersects with the rising alerting system, approximately 2.5 hours after our lowest core body temperature. It is difficult to sleep when core body temperature is rising, a problem experienced by night shift workers who try to sleep during the day. It is almost impossible to initiate sleep during the few hours before our core body temperature begins to fall, when alerting systems are most active.

The *delayed sleep phase type* arises primarily from a history of delay in the timing of the major sleep period (usually more than 2 hours) in relation to the desired sleep and wakeup times, resulting in insomnia and excessive sleepiness. Symptoms include sleep-onset insomnia, difficulty waking in the morning, and excessive early-day sleepiness. People with this pattern are "night owls" who are most alert at night and have difficulty waking in the morning. On the other hand, individuals with the *advanced sleep phase type* are "morning people" who prefer the early morning; their circadian biomarkers, such as melatonin levels and core body temperature rhythms, are "set" 2–4 hours earlier than usual.

DSM-5 also specifies an irregular sleep-wake type and a non-24-hour sleep-wake type.

The *shift work type* of the disorder affects people with unconventional work hours that interfere with maintaining a normal sleep-wake schedule (e.g., night shift workers or people who frequently change their work shift, such as nurses). Shift workers often have high rates of on-the-job sleepiness, tend to make more cognitive errors, and have high rates of drug use and divorce. They might never feel fully rested. The best way to avoid these problems is to forgo shift work, but this may not be possible for some workers. The drug armodafinil (Nuvigil), a stimulant, is FDA-approved for use in people with excessive sleepiness attributed to "shift work disorder" to improve wakefulness.

Parasomnias

Parasomnias are disorders characterized by abnormal behavioral, experiential, or physiological events occurring in association with sleep, specific sleep stages, or sleep-wake transitions.

Non–Rapid Eye Movement Sleep Arousal Disorders

Sleepwalking and sleep terrors—the conditions making up the *non–rapid eye movement sleep arousal disorders*—represent variations of the simultaneous mixture of features of wakefulness and NREM sleep, thereby resulting in appearance of complex motor behavior without conscious awareness (sometimes called "state dissociation").

Sleepwalking consists of episodes of arising from sleep and walking about, usually occurring in the first third of the sleep episode. The patient typically has a blank stare and is relatively unresponsive to others' efforts to communicate; he or she can only be awakened with great difficulty. On waking up, the person has amnesia about the episode and is alert and oriented within minutes. Sleepwalking and sleep terrors generally occur within 3 hours of falling asleep. Electroencephalographic recordings show high-amplitude slow waves preceding the muscular activation that triggers the attack; sleepwalking occurs during Stage 3 NREM sleep.

Sleepwalking episodes usually are brief (<10 minutes). People walk about without purpose and are indifferent to their environment. The disorder is more common in children than adults. Nearly 15% of children have had at least one episode of sleepwalking, but most will outgrow it by late adolescence. In adults, sleepwalking frequently is associated with the presence of a psychiatric disorder, such as major depressive disorder. From 2%–4% of adults have a postchildhood history of sleepwalking.

Sleep terrors—also known as *night terrors*—are a sudden partial arousal from delta sleep associated with screaming and frantic motor activity. These episodes occur during the first third of the sleep episode and often begin with a terrifying scream followed by intense anxiety and signs of autonomic hyperarousal (e.g., rapid breathing). Persons with sleep terrors might not fully awaken after an episode and usually have no detailed recall of the event the next morning. Sleep terrors are uncommon and affect less than 3% of children. The cause of sleep terrors is unknown, but, as with sleepwalking, appear to be familial. Most cases resolve by late adolescence.

Benzodiazepines could help alleviate sleepwalking or sleep terrors through their suppression of Stage 3 sleep. Relapse is likely when the drugs are discontinued or during times of stress. Tricyclic antidepressants, selective serotonin reuptake inhibitors (SSRIs), and melatonin could be effective. Improved sleep hygiene may help in milder cases.

Nightmare Disorder

Nightmare disorder consists of repeated extended, extremely dysphoric, and well-remembered dreams that usually involve efforts to avoid threats to survival, security, or physical integrity. Nightmares can be lengthy and elaborate, with dream imagery that seems real inciting anxiety, fear, or other negative emotions. These generally occur during the second half of the sleep period. On awakening, the individual rapidly becomes alert and oriented. Mild autonomic arousal, including sweating, tachycardia, and tachypnea, could characterize the nightmares, but body movements and vocalizations are not typical. This condition might affect up to 6% of the general population and could become chronic.

Nightmares tend to occur during REM sleep and could emerge at any time during the night, but they are more frequent during the second half, when REM cycles have increased frequency and duration. In childhood, nightmares often are related to specific developmental phases and are particularly common during preschool and early school years. At that age, children may be unable to distinguish reality from dream content.

Nightmares also have been associated with febrile illness and delirium, particularly in elderly and chronically ill persons. Withdrawal from specific drugs, such as the benzodiazepines, also can cause nightmares. More recently, use of SSRIs (e.g., paroxetine, sertraline) and their withdrawal have been linked to vivid dreams or nightmares.

If the nightmares are associated with posttraumatic stress disorder, they could respond to treatment with prazosin. For other types of nightmares, image rehearsal therapy, a form of cognitive-behavioral therapy, is recommended. Relaxation training can also be helpful.

Rapid Eye Movement Sleep Behavior Disorder

Rapid eye movement sleep behavior disorder is defined by the presence of arousal during sleep associated with vocalization and/or complex motor behaviors. The disorder can cause dramatic and potentially violent or injurious behavior arising from REM sleep. The vocalizations often are loud, emotion-filled, and profane. Behaviors may be very bothersome to the individual and the bed partner. REM sleep behavior disorder occurs in less than 1% of the general population but is more prevalent among psychiatric populations. Use of tricyclic antidepressants, SSRIs, serotonin-norepinephrine reuptake inhibitors, and beta-blockers have been associated with REM sleep behavior disorders.

Clonazepam can be effective in treating the disorder, but symptoms promptly return when the medication is discontinued. At least in the short term, the dreamer and the bed partner should be protected by sleeping in different rooms.

Restless Legs Syndrome

Restless legs syndrome, new to DSM-5, is a sensorimotor, neurological sleep disorder characterized by a desire to move the legs, usually associated with uncomfortable sensations typically described as creeping, crawling, tingling, burning, or itching. Symptoms are worse when the individual is at rest, and frequent leg movements occur in an effort to relieve the uncomfortable sensations. Symptoms are worse in the evening or night and in some individuals occur only during those times. Restless legs syndrome is considered a sleep-wake disorder because it interferes with sleep and could be associated with periodic limb movements during sleep.

There are now four FDA-approved medications for restless legs: pramipexole, ropinirole, rotigotine, and gabapentin enacarbil (a prodrug of gabapentin).

Clinical Points for Sleep-Wake Disorders

- A thorough sleep history is essential for accurate diagnosis and includes

  - Drug use patterns.

  - Use of alcohol, caffeine, and stimulant drugs.

  - An interview with the patient's bed partner.

- For patients with insomnia, the sleep hygiene measures are the simplest and most overlooked strategy.

- Be alert to complaints of disturbed sleep, which may point to the possibility of a major psychiatric illness.

  - Major depressive disorder and alcohol use disorders are the most common causes of disturbed sleep.

- Prescribing hypnotics for patients with sleep complaints is inappropriate without first establishing a diagnosis. For insomnia disorder, inform patients that the sleeping pills are for temporary use only (e.g., days to weeks).

- Temazepam and estazolam likely have the best therapeutic properties for a benzodiazepine hypnotic: rapid absorption, lack of metabolites, and an intermediate half-life that will allow a full night's sleep. Nonbenzodiazepine hypnotics are excellent alternatives.

- Some clinicians consider methylphenidate the drug of choice for patients with narcolepsy or hypersomnolence disorder. The dosage should be titrated up to 60 mg/day. Keep track of pill use because some patients may be tempted to abuse this medication. Modafinil is an effective alternative.

- Sodium oxybate is an option for treating narcolepsy complicated by cataplexy.

- If patients have unusual sleep complaints or disorders, make a referral to a sleep disorders clinic for a more thorough evaluation, which may include polysomnography and the Multiple Sleep Latency Test.

Further Reading

American Academy of Sleep Medicine: International Classification of Sleep Disorders, 2nd Edition: Diagnostic and Coding Manual. Westchester, IL, American Academy of Sleep Medicine, 2005

Arnulf I: REM sleep behavior disorder: motor manifestations and pathophysiology. Mov Disord 27(6):677–689, 2012

Aurora RN, Zak RS, Auerbach SH, et al: Best practice guide for the treatment of nightmare disorder in adults. J Clin Sleep Med 6(4):389–401, 2010

Bootzin RR, Epstein DR: Understanding and treating insomnia. Annu Rev Clin Psychol 7:435–458, 2011

Goldsmith RJ, Casola PG: An overview of sleep, sleep disorders, and psychiatric medications' effects on sleep. Psychiatr Ann 36:833–840, 2006

Lam SP, Fong SY, Ho CKW, et al: Parasomnia among psychiatric outpatients: a clinical, epidemiologic, cross-sectional study. J Clin Psychiatry 69(9):1374–1382, 2008

Moser D, Anderer P, Gruber G, et al: Sleep classification according to AASM and Rechtschaffen & Kales: effects on sleep scoring parameters. Sleep 32(2):139–149, 2009

Peterson MJ, Rumble ME, Benca RM: Insomnia and psychiatric disorders. Psychiatr Ann 38:597–605, 2008

Ruoff CM, Reaven NL, Funk SE, et al: High rates of psychiatric comorbidity in narcolepsy: findings from the Burden of Narcolepsy Disease (BOND) Study of 9,312 patients in the United States. J Clin Psychiatry 78(2):171–176, 2017

Zee PC, Lu BS: Insomnia and circadian rhythm sleep disorders. Psychiatr Ann 38:583–589, 2008

Chapter 13

Sexual Dysfunction, Gender Dysphoria, and Paraphilias

Sexual dysfunctions are characterized by disturbance in sexual functioning or desire. *Gender dysphoria* refers to problems in one's sense of maleness or femaleness. *Paraphilic disorders* involve unusual sexual preferences. In DSM-5, each of these diagnostic classes has its own chapter, but the classes are grouped together here for convenience.

Sexual Dysfunctions

Sexual dysfunctions interfere with sexual interest, arousal, or functioning and are surprisingly common. One survey reported prevalence of 38% among women and 29% among men in North America (Table 13–1). These conditions remain "off the radar" because few patients report them to their physicians and even fewer seek treatment.

DSM-5 requires that disorder-specific symptoms (e.g., delayed ejaculation) persist 6 months or longer and that the disorder cause clinically significant distress. Further, the disorder is not due to severe relationship stress; another nonsexual mental disorder; or the effects of a substance, medication, or medical condition (e.g., diabetes mellitus). The clinician can specify whether the symptoms are *lifelong* or *acquired*. If lifelong, the symptoms have been present since the individual became sexually active. Further, the clinician can specify whether the disorder is *generalized* or *situational*. If generalized, the disorder is not limited to specific types of stimulation, situations, or partners.

TABLE 13–1. Frequency of self-reported sexual problems in North American men and women ages 40 to 80 years

Sexual dysfunction	%
Women	
Lack of sexual interest	33
Lubrication difficulties	27
Inability to reach orgasm	25
Pain during sex	14
Men	
Early ejaculation	27
Erectile difficulties	21
Lack of sexual interest	18
Inability to reach orgasm	15

Source.   Adapted from Laumann EO, Nicolosi A, Glasser DB, et al.; GSSAB Investigators' Group: "Sexual Problems Among Women and Men Aged 40–80 y: Prevalence and Correlates Identified in the Global Study of Sexual Attitudes and Behaviors." *International Journal of Impotence Research* 17(1):39–57, 2005.

Dysfunctions

Delayed Ejaculation

Delayed ejaculation occurs when a man achieves ejaculation during sexual activity with great difficulty, if at all, despite adequate stimulation. This usually concerns partnered sexual activity, not masturbation. Some men might avoid sexual activity because of the frustration caused by their difficulty with ejaculation. Typically, the man and his partner report prolonged thrusting to the point of exhaustion or genital discomfort. Some sexual partners might feel responsible for the difficulty and blame themselves (i.e., for not being sufficiently attractive).

Erectile Disorder

Erectile disorder occurs when a man is unable to achieve an erection during partnered sexual activity. The disorder is relatively common, particularly among older men. Erectile disorder is associated with low self-esteem, low self-confidence, and a compromised sense of masculinity. Acquired erectile disorder often is associated with medical factors, such as diabetes and cardiovascular disease, and is likely to be persistent.

Female Orgasmic Disorder

With female orgasmic disorder, the experience of orgasm is diminished, delayed, or even absent on almost all occasions of sexual activity. The disorder sometimes is difficult to assess because women's perceptions of orgasm vary greatly. Many women require clitoral stimulation to reach orgasm, and relatively few report that they always experience orgasm during penile-vaginal intercourse. It is important to consider whether orgasmic difficulties are the result of inadequate sexual stimulation; in these cases, a diagnosis of female orgasmic disorder is not made. Orgasmic difficulties in women often co-occur with problems related to sexual interest and arousal.

Female Sexual Interest/Arousal Disorder

With female sexual interest/arousal disorder, the woman has either a lack of interest in sexual activity or absent/reduced arousal. The disorder occurs in up to one-third of all married women and is defined as the partial or complete failure to attain or maintain the lubrication-swelling response characteristic of the excitement stage or the complete lack of sexual excitement and pleasure. Women with this condition may experience painful intercourse, sexual avoidance, and disturbance of marital or sexual relationships. Temporary low sexual interest can result from stressful situations such as overwork or lack of privacy. Women who are victims of domestic abuse also may report low sexual interest or arousal.

Genito-Pelvic Pain/Penetration Disorder

Genito-pelvic pain/penetration disorder is diagnosed when a woman has pain or discomfort, muscular tightening, or fear about pain when having sexual intercourse. This categorization reflects a change from DSM-IV, whereby two disorders—dyspareunia and vaginismus—were merged into a single category because clinicians had difficulty distinguishing the two. Women experiencing superficial pain during sexual intercourse often have a history of vaginal infections, although pain may persist after successful treatment. Pain during tampon insertion or the inability to insert tampons before any sexual contact has been attempted is an important risk factor for genito-pelvic pain/penetration disorder.

Male Hypoactive Sexual Desire Disorder

Male hypoactive sexual desire disorder is diagnosed when a man has diminished desire for sexual activity and few if any sexual thoughts or fantasies. The disorder could co-occur with erectile problems or abnormal ejaculation. In some, persistent difficulties obtaining an erection can lead the man to lose interest in sexual activity. Men with this disorder often report that they no longer initiate sexual activity and are minimally receptive to a partner's attempt to initiate sexual activity.

Premature (Early) Ejaculation

Premature (early) ejaculation occurs when a man ejaculates during partnered sexual activity within approximately 1 minute after vaginal penetration and before the individual wishes it. Many men with this condition report a sense of lack of control over ejaculation and are apprehensive about their anticipated inability to delay ejaculation during future sexual encounters.

For many, premature (early) ejaculation starts during the man's initial sexual experiences and persists throughout life. In contrast, some men develop the disorder after a period of normal ejaculatory latency, a condition known as *acquired premature (early) ejaculation*. The acquired form likely has a later onset, usually appearing during or after the fourth decade of life.

Substance/Medication-Induced Sexual Dysfunction

Substance/medication-induced sexual dysfunction applies when the effects of a medication or drug of abuse cause clinically significant sexual dysfunction. Acute intoxication or chronic abuse of substances (e.g., cocaine, opiates, amphetamines, sedatives, hypnotics) might decrease sexual interest, cause arousal difficulties, or interfere with orgasm. Many medications (e.g., antihypertensives, histamine H_2 receptor antagonists, antidepressants, anabolic steroids, stimulants, anxiolytics) can lead to sexual dysfunction.

TABLE 13–2. Causes of erectile disorder

Medical illness	Psychiatric illness
Acromegaly	Anxiety disorders
Addison's disease	Dementia
Diabetes	Major depressive disorder
Hyperthyroidism	Schizophrenia
Hypothyroidism	
Klinefelter's syndrome	**Drugs**
Multiple sclerosis	Alcohol
Parkinson's disease	Antiandrogens
Pelvic surgery or irradiation	Anticholinergics
Peripheral vascular disease	Antidepressants
Pituitary adenoma	Antihypertensives (especially centrally acting ones)
Spinal cord injury	
Syphilis	Antipsychotics
Temporal lobe epilepsy	Barbiturates
	Finasteride
	Marijuana
	Opioids
	Stimulants

Causes of Sexual Dysfunction

Sexual dysfunction can be caused by psychological factors, medical conditions, medications, substances of abuse, or, as often happens, a combination of factors.

Up to 75% of the men evaluated for erectile dysfunction have a medical cause for the disorder (Table 13–2). Because medications are so effective in treating erectile disorder, there is little reason for an extensive workup. A limited investigation should include fasting blood glucose to rule out diabetes, and a fasting lipid screen, because erectile dysfunction is a known marker for cardiovascular disease. Some experts also recommend thyroid function tests to rule out hypo- or hyperthyroidism. Obtaining a serum testosterone level might be helpful in some patients to rule out hypogonadism. Specialized tests can be helpful when treatment fails (e.g., Doppler ultrasonography of the penile vasculature, penile angiography).

Differentiate delayed ejaculation from *retrograde ejaculation*, in which ejaculation occurs but the seminal fluid passes backward into the bladder. Both delayed ejaculation and retrograde ejaculation can have a physiological cause, such as the effects of medication, prostatectomy, or neurological disorders involving the lumbosacral section of the spinal cord. Centrally acting antihypertensives, tricyclic antidepressants, or antipsychotics can be responsible for the disorder.

Antidepressants are a frequent cause of sexual dysfunction and could be responsible for low libido, orgasmic disorders in women, and ejaculation delay or failure in men. Up to 65% of persons taking a selective serotonin reuptake inhibitor (SSRI) report some degree of sexual dysfunction. In men, they can cause ejaculatory delay or failure.

Clinical Management

Masters and Johnson developed *brief dual sex therapy*, an approach still widely employed that usually is combined with cognitive-behavioral therapy to correct irrational beliefs and dysfunctional thoughts held by one or both partners. Treatment includes education about normal sexual functioning, graded assignments for specific sexual activities that the couple is expected to carry out in private, and *sensate focus* exercises (i.e., nongenital caressing) to gradually increase awareness of the couple's erogenous zones. These methods can be used for many sexual dysfunctions and are modified depending on the presenting complaint. Other approaches could include the following:

- *Hegar dilators*, which are inserted in the vagina to gradually relieve muscular tightening that occurs with vaginismus.
- The *squeeze method* to halt impending ejaculation to treat premature (early) ejaculation.

Medication now has a large role in treating sexual dysfunctions. SSRIs can be used off-label for premature (early) ejaculation because a common adverse effect of these medications is ejaculatory delay (e.g., paroxetine, 20 mg/day). Men also can benefit from 1% dibucaine (Nupercaine) ointment applied to the coronal ridge and frenulum of the penis to reduce stimulation. Flibanserin has been approved by the FDA to treat premenopausal women with hypoactive sexual desire disorder. Testosterone also has been used to treat men and women with low sexual desire, although research on its use is inconsistent except in clear cases of hypogonadism.

Sildenafil, vardenafil, and tadalafil—FDA-approved to treat erectile disorder—are phosphodiesterase-5 inhibitors that enhance the effect of nitric oxide, which relaxes smooth muscles in the penis, increasing blood flow and allowing an erection to develop in response to sexual arousal. Each of these medications can cause headaches, upset stomach, nausea, and muscle aches. Alprostadil, a synthetic version of the hormone prostaglandin E, is another FDA-approved drug for treating erectile disorder. The drug either is injected directly into the base or side of the penis or is placed directly into the urethra with a special syringe. Surgical treatments of erectile disorder are available, but these are indicated only when medication is ineffective. A simple alternative is a vacuum pump device that produces an erection by increasing blood flow to the penis.

Clinical Points for Sexual Dysfunctions

- Learn to take a sexual history without shame or embarrassment. Patients will detect your anxiety, which will increase their own.

- Do not apologize for asking intimate questions. How a person behaves sexually is important to assess.

  - Most people will be surprisingly forthcoming when describing their sex lives.

- Couples and individuals can engage in sex therapy. The therapy might be used with equal success in opposite- and same-sex couples.

  - The principles of sex therapy are relatively simple to learn and emphasize education about sexual functioning, helping couples to communicate better, and correcting dysfunctional attitudes about sex that one or both partners may hold.

  - Therapy involves homework assignments, which assist the couple in learning to increase sensory awareness. This may include masturbation, sensate focus exercises, and special coital techniques or positions.

- This therapy might help the couple learn to separate pleasure from physiological response (e.g., erection).

- Erectile disorder can be effectively treated pharmacologically, whether the disorder is psychological or medically based. Oral medications include sildenafil, vardenafil, and tadalafil. Another drug, alprostadil, is placed into the urethra with a special applicator or is injected directly into the penis.

  - Surgical techniques are available and involve placing a semi-rigid or an inflatable device.

  - Vacuum pump devices that draw blood into the penis are available.

Gender Dysphoria

Gender dysphoria refers to the distress that can accompany individuals' sense of incongruence between their experience of gender and their assigned gender. In DSM-5, there are separate criteria for children and adolescents/adults. Gender dysphoria has an estimated prevalence of 1 in 30,000 men and 1 in 100,000 women. The disorder usually begins in childhood. In boys, early features include overidentification with the mother, overtly feminine behavior (e.g., playing with dolls), little interest in typical male pursuits (e.g., disliking sports), and peer relationships primarily with girls. Girls might show tomboyish behavior, but this draws little attention from parents because it is more acceptable in our society.

The symptoms of gender dysphoria vary with age. A very young child might show signs of distress (e.g., intense crying) only when parents tell the child that he or she is not "really" a member of the other gender. Adolescents and adults are much more likely to experience distress, but this tends to be mitigated by supportive family and friends. Impairment can vary from school refusal in children to avoiding social activities in adolescents and adults. Depression, anxiety, and substance use disorders can result from gender dysphoria.

When a diagnosis is being made, it is important to rule out other potential causes of gender dysphoria. For example, a desire to change one's anatomical gender might be part of a complex delusion in a person with schizophrenia. DSM-5 subtypes gender dysphoria on the basis of whether the individual has a disorder of sex development (e.g., congenital adrenal disorder, androgen sensitivity syndrome). The clinician also can specify whether the person has transitioned to living full-time in the desired gender ("posttransition").

Many persons with gender dysphoria seek hormonal therapy and gender reassignment surgery. In the transition from male to female, the individual is prescribed hormones (e.g., estradiol, progesterone) to promote development of secondary female characteristics, including breast development. Laser treatment and electrolysis are used to remove hair. Individuals could elect to have surgery to remove the testes and penis and create an artificial vagina (vaginoplasty). A female-to-male patient can elect to undergo mastectomy, hysterectomy, and oophorectomy. Testosterone will help develop muscle mass and deepen the voice. Some persons will choose to have an artificial penis constructed.

Paraphilic Disorders

Paraphilias are defined as involving "anomalous" sexual activity preferences and, in lay terms, include deviant patterns of sexual interests, fantasies, and behaviors. DSM-5 distinguishes between *paraphilia*—the preferred sexual interest—and *paraphilic disorder*—the disorder that can result from the anomalous interest. The diagnosis of a paraphilic disorder requires that, in addition to having a "recurrent and intense sexual arousal" from the anomalous preference, the person has acted on the urges and the urges have caused significant distress or impairment in social, occupational, or other important areas of functioning—or, in the case of pedophilic disorder, "marked distress or interpersonal difficulty." The fantasies, urges, or behaviors must have lasted 6 months or more.

The prevalence of paraphilic disorders is unknown, but isolated incidences of exhibitionism or voyeurism were reported in 3% and 7% of the general population in Sweden, respectively. These disorders are relatively uncommon in psychiatric practice, and most cases come to attention only if the patient seeks treatment or if there are forensic considerations after an arrest (e.g., the person requires evaluation of competency).

Clinical Findings

Paraphilic disorders generally are established in adolescence, usually before age 18. They occur almost exclusively among men, although they can occur in women. Co-occurring psychiatric disorders are common and include substance use disorders, mood and anxiety disorders, and personality disorders. Paraphilic disorders tend to be chronic but vary in frequency of expression and severity depending on the individual's level of stress, opportunity for sexual activity, and sexual drive. Because sexual drive subsides with increasing age, these disorders are probably less common among older adults. DSM-5 paraphilic disorders include the following:

- *Voyeuristic disorder*, which involves looking at or observing ("peeping") unsuspecting persons, usually strangers, who are naked, disrobing, or are engaging in sexual activity.
- *Exhibitionistic disorder*, which involves exposing one's genitals to an unsuspecting person. This disorder accounts for approximately one-third of sexual offenders referred for treatment.
- *Frotteuristic disorder*, which involves touching or rubbing one's genitals against a nonconsenting person.
- *Sexual masochism disorder*, involves sexual fantasies, urges, or behaviors of being humiliated, bound, or otherwise made to suffer that cause clinically significant distress or impairment in social, occupational, or other important areas of functioning.
- *Sexual sadism disorder*, which involves sexual fantasies, urges, or behaviors in which psychological or physical suffering (including humiliation) of a victim is sexually arousing to the person.
- *Pedophilic disorder*, which involves sexual activity with a prepubescent child, generally age 13 or younger. By definition, the individual with pedophilic disorder must be age 16 years or older and at least 5 years older than the child.
- *Fetishistic disorder*, which involves sexual arousal by nonliving objects (e.g., rubber garments, women's underclothing) or a highly specific focus on a nongenital body part (e.g., feet).
- *Transvestic disorder*, which involves cross-dressing that typically begins at puberty. The diagnosis is no longer limited to men as it was in DSM-IV.

Clinical Management of Paraphilic Disorders

Cognitive-behavioral therapy has been used to help restructure the faulty cognitions that people with paraphilic disorders use to justify their behavior. This treatment could be combined with relaxation training to help reduce the anxiety and stress that frequently precede paraphilic behavior. Methods to reduce deviant arousal patterns include *masturbatory satiation* (satiating or boring the patient with his own deviant fantasies) and *covert sensitization* (replacing fantasies with unpleasant images). *Masturbatory conditioning* can be used to help generate arousal to nondeviant themes. Social skills training can help the patient learn to communicate more effectively with appropriate adult partners. Couples therapy can be helpful for those in committed relationships.

There are no FDA-approved medications for paraphilic disorders. SSRIs and naltrexone have been used off-label with some success to reduce deviant fantasies and behaviors. Medroxyprogesterone and leuprolide have been used off-label to reduce serum testosterone levels and to reduce sexual drive.

Clinical Points for Paraphilic Disorders

- The history is of utmost importance in treating paraphilic disorders. Learn where and when the behavior occurs and whether the focus of desire is a person or an object.

  - Most persons with a paraphilic disorder have a variety of deviant sexual interests and behaviors, and the therapist is safe in assuming that more is present than initially meets the eye.

- Paraphilic disorders are challenging to treat, but cognitive-behavioral therapy may offer the best hope for success. The purpose of treatment is to reduce deviant arousal patterns and to generate new arousal patterns to nondeviant themes.

  - Methods could include masturbatory satiation and conditioning, social skills training, and cognitive restructuring.

- Medications could help to reduce paraphilic fantasies and inappropriate sexual behaviors, but none of these medications are FDA-approved for this purpose.

- SSRIs and naltrexone have been used with some success.

- Testosterone-lowering drugs generally are reserved for repeat offenders whose actions are uncontrolled or potentially dangerous.

- In difficult cases, refer the patient to a clinician with experience treating these disorders.

Further Reading

Balon R, Segraves RT (eds): Clinical Manual of Sexual Disorders. Washington, DC, American Psychiatric Publishing, 2009

Balon R, Segraves RT: Sexual dysfunctions, in The American Psychiatric Publishing Textbook of Psychiatry, 6th Edition. Edited by Hales RE, Yudofsky SC, Roberts LW. Washington, DC, American Psychiatric Publishing, 2014, pp 651–678

Becker JV, Perkins A: Gender dysphoria, in The American Psychiatric Publishing Textbook of Psychiatry, 6th Edition. Edited by Hales RE, Yudofsky SC, Roberts LW. Washington, DC, American Psychiatric Publishing, 2014, pp 679–702

Becker JV, Johnson BR, Perkins A: Paraphilic disorders, in The American Psychiatric Publishing Textbook of Psychiatry, 6th Edition. Edited by Hales RE, Yudofsky SC, Roberts LW. Washington, DC, American Psychiatric Publishing, 2014, pp 895–928

Briken P, Kafka MP: Pharmacological treatments for paraphilic patients and sexual offenders. Curr Opin Psychiatry 20(6):609–613, 2007

Grant JE: Clinical characteristics and psychiatric comorbidity in males with exhibitionism. J Clin Psychiatry 66(11):1367–1371, 2005

Hall RC, Hall RC: A profile of pedophilia: definition, characteristics of offenders, recidivism, treatment outcomes, and forensic issues. Mayo Clin Proc 82(4):457–471, 2007

Laumann EO, Nicolosi A, Glasser DB, et al; GSSAB Investigators' Group: Sexual problems among women and men aged 40-80 y: prevalence and correlates identified in the Global Study of Sexual Attitudes and Behaviors. Int J Impot Res 17(1):39–57, 2005

Morrison SD, Chen ML, Crane CN: An overview of female-to-male gender-confirming surgery. Nat Rev Urol 14(8):486–500, 2017

Schiavi RC, Schreiner-Engel P, Mandeli J, et al: Healthy aging and male sexual function. Am J Psychiatry 147(6):766–771, 1990

Disruptive, Impulse-Control, and Conduct Disorders

Impaired self-regulation is the hallmark of disruptive, impulse-control, and conduct disorders. These disorders are associated with physical or verbal injury to self, others, or objects or with violating the rights of others. Although common, they are frequently underappreciated and ignored. The DSM-5 disruptive, impulse-control, and conduct disorders are listed in Table 14–1.

Oppositional Defiant Disorder

Oppositional defiant disorder (ODD) is a diagnosis for children and adolescents with difficult but not generally dangerous or illegal behaviors. The DSM-5 criteria for oppositional defiant disorder are shown in Box 14–1.

Box 14–1.   DSM-5 Criteria for Oppositional
            Defiant Disorder

A. A pattern of angry/irritable mood, argumentative/defiant behavior, or vindictiveness lasting at least 6 months as evidenced by at least four symptoms from any of the following categories, and exhibited during interaction with at least one individual who is not a sibling.

Angry/Irritable Mood

1. Often loses temper.
2. Is often touchy or easily annoyed.
3. Is often angry and resentful.

Argumentative/Defiant Behavior

4. Often argues with authority figures or, for children and adolescents, with adults.

5. Often actively defies or refuses to comply with requests from authority figures or with rules.
6. Often deliberately annoys others.
7. Often blames others for his or her mistakes or misbehavior.

Vindictiveness

8. Has been spiteful or vindictive at least twice within the past 6 months.

Note: The persistence and frequency of these behaviors should be used to distinguish a behavior that is within normal limits from a behavior that is symptomatic. For children younger than 5 years, the behavior should occur on most days for a period of at least 6 months unless otherwise noted (Criterion A8). For individuals 5 years or older, the behavior should occur at least once per week for at least 6 months, unless otherwise noted (Criterion A8). While these frequency criteria provide guidance on a minimal level of frequency to define symptoms, other factors should also be considered, such as whether the frequency and intensity of the behaviors are outside a range that is normative for the individual's developmental level, gender, and culture.

B. The disturbance in behavior is associated with distress in the individual or others in his or her immediate social context (e.g., family, peer group, work colleagues), or it impacts negatively on social, educational, occupational, or other important areas of functioning.
C. The behaviors do not occur exclusively during the course of a psychotic, substance use, depressive, or bipolar disorder. Also, the criteria are not met for disruptive mood dysregulation disorder.

TABLE 14–1. DSM-5 disruptive, impulse-control, and conduct disorders

---

Oppositional defiant disorder

Intermittent explosive disorder

Conduct disorder

Antisocial personality disorder (criteria included with the personality disorders [see Chapter 17 in this guide])

Pyromania

Kleptomania

ODD has a prevalence of approximately 3%, and before adolescence it is more frequent in boys. The gender ratio appears to equal out after puberty. ODD first appears during the preschool years and rarely later and could precede onset of conduct disorder. Children and adolescents with ODD are at risk for mood and anxiety disorders. Rule out other disorders, including conduct disorder, attention-deficit/hyperactivity disorder (ADHD), disruptive mood dysregulation disorder, and intermittent explosive disorder.

Treating ODD emphasizes individual and family counseling while treating co-occurring ADHD or other disorders with appropriate medications. Cognitive-behavioral therapy (CBT) can help the child manage anger, improve problem-solving ability, develop techniques to delay impulsive responses, and improve social interactions. With parental management training, parents learn to better manage their child's behavior as well as promote desired behaviors.

Intermittent Explosive Disorder

Intermittent explosive disorder (IED) is diagnosed when a person has verbal aggression or behavioral outbursts representing a failure to control aggressive impulses. These episodes are out of proportion to the provocation or the psychosocial stressor. The diagnosis is used for persons whose loss of control is out of character and not merely part of a pattern of overreacting to life's problems. Therefore, rule out mental disorders in which assaultive behaviors occur as a matter of course, such as antisocial or borderline personality disorders, psychotic disorders, mania, or alcohol or drug use disorders. A sudden behavioral change accompanied by outbursts in an otherwise healthy person suggests a neurocognitive disorder, which also should be ruled out. The DSM-5 criteria for IED are shown in Box 14–2.

Box 14–2.   Intermittent Explosive Disorder

A. Recurrent behavioral outbursts representing a failure to control aggressive impulses as manifested by either of the following:

1. Verbal aggression (e.g., temper tantrums, tirades, verbal arguments or fights) or physical aggression toward property, animals, or other individuals, occurring twice weekly,

on average, for a period of 3 months. The physical aggression does not result in damage or destruction of property and does not result in physical injury to animals or other individuals.

2. Three behavioral outbursts involving damage or destruction of property and/or physical assault involving physical injury against animals or other individuals occurring within a 12-month period.

B. The magnitude of aggressiveness expressed during the recurrent outbursts is grossly out of proportion to the provocation or to any precipitating psychosocial stressors.

C. The recurrent aggressive outbursts are not premeditated (i.e., they are impulsive and/or anger-based) and are not committed to achieve some tangible objective (e.g., money, power, intimidation).

D. The recurrent aggressive outbursts cause either marked distress in the individual or impairment in occupational or interpersonal functioning, or are associated with financial or legal consequences.

E. Chronological age is at least 6 years (or equivalent developmental level).

F. The recurrent aggressive outbursts are not better explained by another mental disorder (e.g., major depressive disorder, bipolar disorder, disruptive mood dysregulation disorder, a psychotic disorder, antisocial personality disorder, borderline personality disorder) and are not attributable to another medical condition (e.g., head trauma, Alzheimer's disease) or to the physiological effects of a substance (e.g., a drug of abuse, a medication). For children ages 6–18 years, aggressive behavior that occurs as part of an adjustment disorder should not be considered for this diagnosis.

Individuals with IED primarily are young men with relatively low frustration tolerance. A recent study found a 7% lifetime prevalence, but some experts suggest that "pure" cases of IED—that is, cases unaccompanied by any indication of a brain disorder (e.g., abnormal electroencephalographic findings, neurological soft signs) or a personality disorder—are rare.

Medication to treat aggressive impulses can be helpful, although none are FDA-approved. The selective serotonin reuptake inhibitor (SSRI) fluoxetine and the antiepileptic drug oxcarbazepine appear effective in reducing impulsive aggression in individuals with IED. Other SSRIs, mood stabilizers, and beta-blockers have been used to treat IED, but their role is unclear. Second-generation antipsychotics have been employed to dampen aggressive impulses in other clinical populations (e.g., dementia patients, people with borderline personality disorder) and might be helpful in the treatment of IED. Avoid benzodiazepines because of their tendency to cause behavioral disinhibition.

CBT could help patients learn to recognize when they are becoming angry and identify and defuse the triggers that lead to outbursts.

Conduct Disorder

Conduct disorder is a pattern of recurrent behavioral problems in children or adolescents that is a forerunner of antisocial personality disorder in adults. DSM-5 criteria require the presence of at least 3 of 15 antisocial behaviors in the past 12 months (with at least 1 criterion present in the past 6 months). The *childhood-onset type* begins before age 10 years and probably has a more guarded prognosis, whereas the *adolescent-onset type* begins after age 10 years and is more likely to have a better outcome. The DSM-5 criteria for conduct disorder are shown in Box 14–3.

Box 14–3. DSM-5 Criteria for Conduct Disorder

A. A repetitive and persistent pattern of behavior in which the basic rights of others or major age-appropriate societal norms or rules are violated, as manifested by the presence of at least three of the following 15 criteria in the past 12 months from any of the categories below, with at least one criterion present in the past 6 months:

Aggression to People and Animals

1. Often bullies, threatens, or intimidates others.
2. Often initiates physical fights.
3. Has used a weapon that can cause serious physical harm to others (e.g., a bat, brick, broken bottle, knife, gun).
4. Has been physically cruel to people.
5. Has been physically cruel to animals.
6. Has stolen while confronting a victim (e.g., mugging, purse snatching, extortion, armed robbery).
7. Has forced someone into sexual activity.

Destruction of Property

8. Has deliberately engaged in fire setting with the intention of causing serious damage.
9. Has deliberately destroyed others' property (other than by fire setting).

Deceitfulness or Theft

10. Has broken into someone else's house, building, or car.
11. Often lies to obtain goods or favors or to avoid obligations (i.e., "cons" others).
12. Has stolen items of nontrivial value without confronting a victim (e.g., shoplifting, but without breaking and entering; forgery).

Serious Violations of Rules

13. Often stays out at night despite parental prohibitions, beginning before age 13 years.
14. Has run away from home overnight at least twice while living in the parental or parental surrogate home, or once without returning for a lengthy period.
15. Is often truant from school, beginning before age 13 years.

B. The disturbance in behavior causes clinically significant impairment in social, academic, or occupational functioning.
C. If the individual is age 18 years or older, criteria are not met for antisocial personality disorder.

Children who are especially difficult can be further designated as having *limited prosocial emotions*. With this subtype, the child exhibits callous behavior and lack of remorse.

Approximately 8% of boys and 3% of girls have a pattern of behaviors that meets criteria for conduct disorder. Research shows that an estimated 40% of boys and 25% of girls with conduct disorder eventually will qualify for an antisocial personality disorder diagnosis. Children who are able to form relationships and internalize social norms have a better outcome, as do children who are less aggressive. Children who develop conduct problems at a very early age (e.g., 5 years) are more likely to have an enduring pattern of antisocial behavior than children who develop behavioral problems linked to teenage peer pressure. Conduct disorder is highly comorbid with ADHD, mood and anxiety disorders, and specific learning disorders.

Treatment recommendations vary depending on the age of the child, symptom severity, comorbidity, family supports, and the child's intellectual and social assets. A relatively mild case typically is treated with individual and family therapy. At the opposite end of the spectrum are those cases in which the child comes from a highly deviant family and engages in repeated antisocial acts that bring him or her to legal attention. In these cases, the child may need to be removed from the home and placed in a group home or juvenile detention facility. Parental management training can be an important part of managing the child's behavior. This training involves teaching parents to communicate more effectively with their child, to apply appropriate and consistent discipline, to monitor the child's whereabouts, and to steer the child away from bad peers.

Medication should target co-occurring disorders (e.g., ADHD). Lithium, psychostimulants, haloperidol, and second-generation antipsychotics sometimes are used off-label to help manage aggression in children with conduct disorder who are out of control.

Pyromania

Pyromania is the deliberate and purposeful setting of fire on more than one occasion. The act is preceded by a feeling of tension or affective arousal, followed by a sense of pleasure, gratification, or relief. Such persons are fascinated by fire. The arsonist who sets fires for monetary gain or for political or criminal purposes does not qualify for the diagnosis. Deliberate fire setting probably is motivated most frequently by anger or revenge.

The disorder is uncommon and mostly occurs in boys and men. Onset tends to be in the late teens or early 20s. Mood disorders, substance use disorders, and other impulsive behaviors are common among people with pyromania.

There is no clear role for medication for treating pyromania. If the patient is a child or adolescent, teach parents consistent but nonpunitive discipline methods. Family therapy can help in dealing with the broader issue of family dysfunction often found in these patients. Educate patients about the dangerousness and significance of fire setting. Patients need to learn alternative ways of coping with stressful situations to decrease reliance on fire setting as an outlet.

Kleptomania

Kleptomania involves the recurrent failure to resist impulses to steal objects not needed for personal use or for their monetary value. Persons with this disorder generally describe an increasing sense of tension immediately before the theft, followed by a sense of pleasure, gratification, or relief. The stealing is not committed to express anger or vengeance, nor does it occur in response to hallucinations or delusions. Antisocial personality disorder, conduct disorder, and mania should be ruled out as a cause of the stealing.

The prevalence of kleptomania is unknown. Mood and anxiety disorders frequently co-occur. Stealing impulses and behaviors often change with the patient's mood. Kleptomania begins in adolescence or early adulthood and tends to be chronic. Nearly three-quarters of persons with kleptomania are women.

SSRIs and naltrexone have been used off-label to reduce a patient's urge to steal. Treating comorbid disorders (e.g., major depressive disorder) also might help reduce the stealing behaviors, particularly if the stealing is prompted by dysphoric moods.

CBT might help steer the individual away from stealing and help him or her avoid cues that trigger stealing. Teach the individual to substitute other, more benign behaviors to replace the stealing (e.g., socializing with friends rather than shopping alone).

Other Disruptive, Impulse-Control, and Conduct Disorders

Compulsive shopping and Internet addiction are two disorders that, although not listed in DSM-5, are problematic and well described in the literature.

Compulsive Shopping

Compulsive shopping is characterized by an irresistible urge to buy items that are unneeded or unwanted. The person usually has a feeling of tension before buying, followed by a sense of gratification or relief with buying. Rule out mania as a cause of the excessive shopping. There is no standard treatment, although CBT may help.

Internet Addiction

Internet addiction involves excessive or poorly controlled computer use that leads to impairment or distress. There is no consensus regarding its treatment, but limiting a person's Internet access may help. *Internet gaming disorder* is a variant of Internet addiction but is focused on those who are preoccupied with computer-based games.

Clinical Points for Disruptive, Impulse-Control, and Conduct Disorders

- ODD must be distinguished from normal defiant behavior that typically occurs in young children (ages 2–4) and adolescents. Treatment will necessarily target both the child and the family.

- IED could respond to the SSRI fluoxetine, a mood stabilizer (e.g., oxcarbazepine), propranolol, or a second-generation antipsychotic.

  - CBT could help patients learn to identify stressors that trigger outbursts, which patients can then defuse.

  - Patients must know that they are responsible for the consequences of their behavior.

- Conduct disorder is very difficult to treat, but in mild cases the patient may respond to a combination of psychotherapy and medication to reduce anger and irritability.

  - Family therapy is essential because parents need help to understand and manage their misbehaving child.

- The child with pyromania might benefit from fire safety training.

- Persons with kleptomania could benefit from naltrexone or an SSRI (e.g., fluoxetine, paroxetine).

  - A self-imposed shopping ban might be the best short-term strategy to forestall stealing.

- The person with Internet addiction who lives at home should have his or her computer access monitored.

  - Parents should consider canceling Internet service or limiting computer use.

Further Reading

Black DW: Bad Boys, Bad Men: Confronting Antisocial Personality Disorder. New York, Oxford University Press, 1999

Black DW: A review of compulsive buying disorder. World Psychiatry 6(1):14–18, 2007

Coccaro EF, Lee RJ, Kavoussi RJ: A double-blind, randomized, placebo-controlled trial of fluoxetine in patients with intermittent explosive disorder. J Clin Psychiatry 70(5):653–662, 2009

Grant JE, Potenza MN (eds): The Oxford Handbook of Impulse Control Disorders. New York, Oxford University Press, 2012

Grant JE, Won Kim S: Clinical characteristics and psychiatric comorbidity of pyromania. J Clin Psychiatry 68(11):1717–1722, 2007

Grant JE, Kim SW, Odlaug BL: A double-blind, placebo-controlled study of the opiate antagonist, naltrexone, in the treatment of kleptomania. Biol Psychiatry 65(7):600–606, 2009

Kolko DJ: Efficacy of cognitive-behavioral treatment and fire safety education for children who set fires: initial and follow-up outcomes. J Child Psychol Psychiatry 42(3):359–369, 2001

Mattes JA: Oxcarbazepine in patients with impulsive aggression: a double-blind, placebo-controlled trial. J Clin Psychopharmacol 25(6):575–579, 2005

McCloskey MS, Noblett KL, Deffenbacher JL, et al: Cognitive-behavioral therapy for intermittent explosive disorder: a pilot randomized clinical trial. J Consult Clin Psychol 76(5):876–886, 2008

Shaw M, Black DW: Internet addiction: definition, assessment, epidemiology and clinical management. CNS Drugs 22(5):353–365, 2008

Chapter 15

Substance-Related and Addictive Disorders

The misuse of alcohol or other drugs is widespread and growing. Nearly two-thirds of adult Americans occasionally drink alcohol, and 12% drink almost every day and become intoxicated several times a month. Marijuana has been used by more than one-quarter of Americans, and nearly 6 million have admitted using cocaine in the prior year. Patterns of use change, however, reflecting the fluctuating popularity of drugs and their availability and cost.

Ten substance-related disorder classes are reviewed in this chapter (see Table 15–1). DSM-IV's pathological gambling, renamed *gambling disorder*, has been moved to this diagnostic class, reflecting evidence that gambling activates the brain's reward system similarly to drugs of abuse. Although the term *addiction* appears in the title of the chapter, it is not used as a diagnostic term in DSM-5.

Substance use disorders follow a set of standard criteria. In each disorder, 2 or more of 11 problematic behaviors must occur within a 12-month period leading to clinically significant impairment or distress. The 11 symptoms involve overall groupings of impaired control, social impairment, risky use, and pharmacological criteria (i.e., evidence of tolerance or withdrawal). **Because these criteria sets are similar, only the criteria set for alcohol use disorder is reproduced in this chapter** (see Box 15–1 in section "Alcohol-Related Disorders" below). In DSM-5, if a patient has signs and symptoms that meet criteria for more than one substance use disorder, all the disorders for which criteria are met are diagnosed.

Substance use disorders are rated for severity: mild requires the presence of two or three symptoms; moderate, four or five symptoms; and severe, six or more symptoms. Clinicians also can specify if the disorder is in "early remission" (i.e., no symptom criteria met for the past 3 months), or "sustained remission" (i.e., no symptom criteria met for the past 12 months).

TABLE 15–1. DSM-5 substance-related and addictive disorders

Alcohol-related disorders	**Opioid-related disorders**
Alcohol use disorder	Opioid use disorder
Alcohol intoxication	Opioid intoxication
Alcohol withdrawal	Opioid withdrawal
Caffeine-related disorders	**Sedative-, hypnotic-, or anxiolytic-related disorders**
Caffeine intoxication	
Caffeine withdrawal	Sedative, hypnotic, or anxiolytic use disorder
Cannabis-related disorders	Sedative, hypnotic, or anxiolytic intoxication
Cannabis use disorder	
Cannabis intoxication	Sedative, hypnotic, or anxiolytic withdrawal
Cannabis withdrawal	**Stimulant-related disorders**
Hallucinogen-related disorders	Stimulant use disorder
Phencyclidine use disorder	Stimulant intoxication
Other hallucinogen use disorder	Stimulant withdrawal
Phencyclidine intoxication	**Tobacco-related disorders**
Other hallucinogen intoxication	Tobacco use disorder
Hallucinogen persisting perception disorder	Tobacco withdrawal
Inhalant-related disorders	**Non-substance-related disorders**
Inhalant use disorder	Gambling disorder
Inhalant intoxication	

Assessment of Substance-Related Disorders

Assessment of substance-related disorders requires a thorough history, physical examination, and mental status examination. Many addicted persons will have co-occurring mental disorders, such as major depressive disorder, bipolar disorder, or an anxiety disorder, that should be diagnosed and treated. Antisocial and borderline personality disorders are common among those who abuse substances.

Collateral history from relatives or friends or from other physicians will help fill in the gaps. Even patients who are straightforward about their misuse of substances might minimize its severity. A physical examination can offer signs of intoxication and withdrawal, depending on when the individual presents at a hospital or clinic.

Laboratory testing for substances of abuse has become a routine part of the workup. Intoxication and overdose are the most common indications to test for drugs of abuse, but consider such testing when assessing a patient who presents with alterations in mood or behavior. Most testing involves sampling blood or urine.

Alcohol-Related Disorders

Alcohol is one of the most commonly abused substances and is associated with significant morbidity and mortality. Although common in the general population, alcohol-related disorders are even more frequent in hospital patients, including 25%–50% of medical-surgical patients and up to 50%–60% of psychiatric inpatients in some settings. There are two to three men for each woman with an alcohol use disorder, and onset is usually between ages 16 and 30. Onset is earlier in men than in women, although the medical complications progress more rapidly in women.

Diagnosis and Assessment

Alcohol use disorder is a problematic pattern of alcohol use leading to clinically significant impairment or distress. Two or more of 11 problematic behaviors must occur within a 12-month period for the diagnosis to be made (Box 15–1). Depending on the number of symptoms present, the disorder is specified as *mild*, *moderate*, or *severe*. Separate categories are used for *alcohol intoxication* and *alcohol withdrawal*. The clinician should record all diagnoses that are present (e.g., alcohol intoxication, moderate alcohol use disorder).

Box 15–1.   DSM-5 Criteria for Alcohol Use
             Disorder[a]

A. A problematic pattern of alcohol use leading to clinically significant impairment or distress, as manifested by at least two of the following, occurring within a 12-month period:

1. Alcohol is often taken in larger amounts or over a longer period than was intended.
2. There is a persistent desire or unsuccessful efforts to cut down or control alcohol use.
3. A great deal of time is spent in activities necessary to obtain alcohol, use alcohol, or recover from its effects.
4. Craving, or a strong desire or urge to use alcohol.
5. Recurrent alcohol use resulting in a failure to fulfill major role obligations at work, school, or home.
6. Continued alcohol use despite having persistent or recurrent social or interpersonal problems caused or exacerbated by the effects of alcohol.
7. Important social, occupational, or recreational activities are given up or reduced because of alcohol use.
8. Recurrent alcohol use in situations in which it is physically hazardous.
9. Alcohol use is continued despite knowledge of having a persistent or recurrent physical or psychological problem that is likely to have been caused or exacerbated by alcohol.
10. Tolerance, as defined by either of the following:
    a. A need for markedly increased amounts of alcohol to achieve intoxication or desired effect.
    b. A markedly diminished effect with continued use of the same amount of alcohol.
11. Withdrawal, as manifested by either of the following:
    a. The characteristic withdrawal syndrome for alcohol (refer to Criteria A and B of the criteria set for alcohol withdrawal).
    b. Alcohol (or a closely related substance, such as a benzodiazepine) is taken to relieve or avoid withdrawal symptoms.

aCriteria for alcohol use disorder are shown to represent the similar criteria sets for all the DSM-5 substance use disorders.

The four-question CAGE test is a simple screen that can assess the presence of an alcohol use disorder (Table 15–2). Problematic use is suggested by any positive response or overly defensive answer.

Blood alcohol concentration roughly correlates with level of intoxication. The following levels apply to persons who are not tolerant to alcohol:

- 0–100 mg/dL: A sense of well-being, sedation, tranquility
- 100–150 mg/dL: Incoordination, irritability

TABLE 15–2. CAGE: screening tool for an alcohol use disorder

C	Have you felt the need to CUT DOWN on your drinking?
A	Have you felt ANNOYED BY CRITICISM of your drinking?
G	Have you felt GUILTY (or had regrets) about your drinking?
E	Have you felt the need for an EYE-OPENER in the morning?

Source. Adapted from Ewing JA: "Detecting Alcoholism. The CAGE Questionnaire." *JAMA* 252(14):1905–1907, 1984.

- 150–250 mg/dL: Slurred speech, ataxia
- >250 mg/dL: Passing out, unconsciousness

Concentrations >350 mg/dL can lead to coma and death. The presence of few clinical symptoms of intoxication in a person with a level of ≥150 mg/dL is strong evidence of an alcohol use disorder.

People with an alcohol use disorder can develop increased high-density lipoprotein cholesterol, increased lactate dehydroxygenase, decreased low-density lipoprotein cholesterol, decreased blood urea nitrogen, decreased red blood cell volume, and increased uric acid level. Mean corpuscular volume is increased in up to 95% of individuals with an alcohol use disorder. Liver enzymes frequently are abnormal, including an increase in γ-glutamyltransferase (GGT) level, which may be an early sign of alcohol misuse. Transaminase (aspartate aminotransferase and alanine aminotransferase) levels also are increased.

Clinical Findings

Early on, alcohol misuse can be difficult to identify. Because of denial, family members and coworkers often are in the best position to identify early symptoms, because they may observe poor work productivity, lateness or unexplained absences, irritability, or moodiness. As the disorder progresses, physical changes can occur: development of acne rosacea; palmar erythema; or painless enlargement of the liver consistent with fatty infiltration. Other early manifestations include respiratory or other infections, unexplained bruises, periods of amnesia, minor accidents (e.g., unexplained falls at home), and concerns about the person's driving skills or an arrest or accident related to driving while intoxicated. As the disorder advances, jaundice or ascites can develop, as can testicular atrophy, gynecomastia, and Dupuytren's contractures. At this point alcohol misuse probably has disrupted the person's life, contributing to job loss, loss of friendships, and marital discord and family problems.

Medical Complications

Alcohol use disorders can affect a person's medical and emotional health and lead to a broad range of social problems (Table 15–3). Medical problems range from benign fatty infiltration of the liver to fulminant liver failure. Almost all organ systems are affected by heavy use of alcohol. The gastrointestinal tract is particularly affected, with consequences including gastritis, diarrhea, and peptic ulcers. Other effects include fatty infiltration of the liver, cirrhosis in approximately 10% of heavy drinkers, and pancreatitis. Cardiomyopathy, thrombocytopenia, anemia, and myopathy all have been reported.

The central nervous system (CNS) and peripheral nervous system could be damaged by the direct and indirect effects of alcohol. Peripheral neuropathy commonly occurs in a stocking-and-glove distribution, probably the result of an alcohol-induced vitamin B deficiency. Cerebellar damage can cause dysarthria and ataxia. Thiamine deficiency could cause Wernicke's encephalopathy and consists of nystagmus, ataxia, and mental confusion, which could reverse with an injection of thiamine. Dementia can develop as a result of vitamin deficiency or the direct effects of alcohol, although the exact mechanism is unknown. Chronic alcohol misuse also has been associated with enlarged cerebral ventricles and widened cortical sulci, effects that might be partially reversible when the individual stops drinking.

The *fetal alcohol syndrome* (FAS) has been described in children whose mothers abuse alcohol while pregnant. This syndrome is related to excessive maternal consumption of alcohol during pregnancy, especially when binge drinking produces a surge in blood alcohol levels. Abnormalities include facial anomalies, low IQ, and behavior problems. FAS affects approximately 1–2 infants per 100,000 live births. Women should be warned that alcohol consumption during pregnancy can cause FAS.

Alcohol consumption is a frequent cause of traumatic injuries and contributes to more than 50% of all motor vehicle

TABLE 15–3. Medical and psychosocial hazards associated with alcohol use disorders

Drug interactions

Gastrointestinal
  Esophageal bleeding
  Mallory-Weiss tear
  Gastritis
  Intestinal malabsorption
Pancreatitis
Liver disease
  Fatty infiltration
  Hepatitis
  Cirrhosis
Nutritional deficiency
  Malnutrition
  Vitamin B deficiency
Neuropsychiatric
  Wernicke-Korsakoff syndrome
  Cortical atrophy/ventricular dilation
  Alcohol-induced dementia
  Peripheral neuropathy
  Myopathy
  Depression
  Suicide
Endocrine system
  Testicular atrophy
  Increased estrogen levels

Alcohol withdrawal
  Uncomplicated withdrawal (the "shakes")
  Seizures
  Hallucinosis
  Withdrawal delirium (delirium tremens)
Infectious disease
  Pneumonia
  Tuberculosis
Cardiovascular
  Cardiomyopathy
  Hypertension
Cancer
  Oral cavity
  Esophagus
  Large intestine/rectum
  Liver
  Pancreas
Birth defects
  Fetal alcohol syndrome
Psychosocial
  Accidents
  Crime
  Spouse and child abuse
  Job loss
  Divorce, separation

deaths each year. Household injuries are common. Subdural hematomas occur in many older persons who fall and sustain head injuries when intoxicated.

Cancer rates of the mouth, tongue, larynx, esophagus, stomach, liver, and pancreas are increased. The precise role that alcohol plays in these cancers is uncertain because its effects are confounded by those of smoking and tobacco use. Alcohol interferes with male sexual function and can cause impotence and affect fertility by lowering serum testosterone levels. Increased circulating levels of estrogen can lead to breast enlargement (gynecomastia) and female escutcheon (pubic hair pattern) in men.

Course and Outcome

In a review of 10 large studies, 2%–3% of people with an alcohol use disorder become abstinent each year, and approximately 1% return to asymptomatic or controlled drinking. These findings were true for both treated and untreated samples, supporting the hypothesis that alcohol use disorders are self-limiting for some persons. In the 10 studies, 46%–87% of the subjects continued to misuse alcohol at follow-up; 0%–33% were asymptomatic drinkers; and 8%–39% had achieved abstinence.

Clinical Management

Treatment of alcohol withdrawal depends on the syndrome that develops. Withdrawal symptoms typically follow abrupt cessation of alcohol consumption *or* when users simply reduce their intake. Mild tremors and nausea are the most common symptoms; far fewer patients will have had seizures, hallucinations, or delirium tremens.

- *Uncomplicated alcohol withdrawal* (the "shakes") begins 12–18 hours after stopping drinking, peaks at 24–48 hours, and subsides within 5–7 days. Symptoms include anxiety, tremors, and nausea and vomiting; heart rate and blood pressure might be increased.
- *Alcoholic withdrawal seizures* ("rum fits") occur 7–38 hours after cessation of drinking and peak between 24 and 48 hours. Withdrawal seizures occur primarily as a consequence of severe, long-term alcohol misuse.
- *Alcoholic hallucinosis*—vivid and unpleasant auditory, visual, or tactile hallucinations—begins within 48 hours of drinking cessation and occurs in the presence of a clear sensorium. Hallucinations are a sign of severe alcohol misuse.
- *Alcohol withdrawal delirium* (delirium tremens, or "DTs") is rare but alarming. Delirium begins 2–3 days after drinking

stops or after a significant reduction of intake and peaks 4–5 days later. Symptoms include confusion, agitation, perceptual disturbance, mild fever, and autonomic hyperarousal. DTs can be fatal.

The management of alcohol withdrawal consists of general support (i.e., adequate food and hydration, careful medical monitoring), nutritional supplementation, and use of benzodiazepines. People with a history of uncomplicated withdrawal can be managed as outpatients. Treatment primarily involves benzodiazepines that, once the patient is comfortable, are tapered gradually. Any benzodiazepine will work, but longer-acting ones (chlordiazepoxide, clonazepam, diazepam) are preferred because they provide a smoother withdrawal course. Those who have comorbid medical disorders, are significantly depressed or suicidal, have impaired ability to follow instructions or poor social support, or have a history of severe withdrawal symptoms might need to be hospitalized.

Patients should receive an adequate diet plus oral thiamine (100 mg), folic acid (1 mg), and multivitamins. Thiamine (100–200 mg intramuscularly) can be administered if oral intake is not possible and should be given before any situation in which glucose loading is required because glucose can deplete thiamine stores. There are two approaches commonly used for dosing benzodiazepines:

- With *symptom-triggered management*, medication is given based on the patient's signs/symptoms of withdrawal (often based on the Clinical Institute Withdrawal Assessment for Alcohol Scale, Revised [CIWA-Ar]). The scale rates nausea and vomiting, tremor, anxiety, and other symptoms of withdrawal. For example, chlordiazepoxide 25 mg might be given orally every 2 hours as needed for a person with a CIWA-Ar score ≥10.
- With *fixed dosing*, medication is given on a predetermined dosing schedule based on the patient's estimated tolerance, supplemented by "as needed" doses. Those at risk for severe withdrawal symptoms might do better with fixed dosing (Table 15–4). Additional doses can be given for breakthrough signs or symptoms (e.g., tremors or diaphoresis). The 10-item CIWA-Ar is an objective rating scale that can be used to monitor the patient's withdrawal state.

TABLE 15–4. Fixed dosing for managing alcohol withdrawal

Chlordiazepoxide protocol

- 50 mg every 4 hours × 24 hours, then
- 50 mg every 6 hours × 24 hours, then
- 25 mg every 4 hours × 24 hours, then
- 25 mg every 6 hours × 24 hours

Some patients will benefit from anti-nausea agents, non-steroidal anti-inflammatory drugs for pain or headache, or loperamide for diarrhea. Delirious patients will need specialized care, while those with frightening hallucinations might benefit from a second-generation antipsychotic.

Rehabilitation

Rehabilitation has two goals: 1) the patient remains sober, and 2) coexisting disorders are identified and treated. Patients with comorbid mood or anxiety disorders will benefit with treatment. Because alcohol use disorder itself can cause depression, and since most alcohol-induced depressions lift with sobriety, antidepressants are needed only for those who remain depressed after 2–4 weeks of sobriety.

Participation in group therapy will enable the patient to see their problems mirrored in others and learn better coping skills. With individual therapy, the person can learn to identify triggers that prompt drinking and learn more effective coping strategies. *Motivational interviewing* increasingly is being used to help persuade patients to make their own case for change (i.e., to abandon alcohol).

Encourage patients to attend Alcoholics Anonymous (AA). Family therapy often is important because the family system that has been altered to accommodate the person's drinking might end up reinforcing it.

Medication

Three drugs are FDA-approved to treat DSM-IV alcohol dependence (which roughly corresponds to DSM-5's moderate or severe alcohol use disorder).

- Disulfiram inhibits aldehyde dehydrogenase, an enzyme necessary for metabolizing alcohol. This results in the accumulation of acetaldehyde when alcohol is consumed. Acetaldehyde is toxic and induces noxious symptoms, such as nausea, vomiting, palpitations, and hypotension. Because patients taking disulfiram are aware of the potential adverse reaction, they are motivated to avoid alcohol.
- Naltrexone, a mu-opioid antagonist, appears to reduce the pleasurable effects of and craving for alcohol. The drug generally is well tolerated but can produce nausea, headache, anxiety, or sedation. A black-box warning advises that naltrexone should not be given to people with severe liver disease and that its use requires periodic monitoring of liver enzymes. Naltrexone is available in a long-acting injectable formulation.
- Acamprosate, a glutamate receptor modulator, also helps curb urges to drink, thereby helping individuals maintain abstinence. Acamprosate is generally well tolerated, but some patients report headache, diarrhea, flatulence, and nausea.

Clinical Points for Management of Alcohol-Related Disorders

- People who misuse alcohol need acceptance and not blame.

- Even if the person has failed to benefit from rehabilitation efforts, do not give up!

- Treatment of alcohol withdrawal should take place in an inpatient setting if the patient has a history of severe "shakes," hallucinations, seizures, or delirium tremens. Other patients—perhaps most—can be treated on an outpatient basis.

  - Any benzodiazepine will work, but longer-acting ones (e.g., chlordiazepoxide, clonazepam, diazepam) are preferred.

- Manage the patient's other comorbid disorders (e.g., major depressive disorder); if untreated, these disorders can contribute to relapse.

- Refer the patient to AA to provide ongoing social support and encouragement from persons similarly affected.

- Include the family in the treatment process.

  - Alcohol use disorders affect every member of the family, and unresolved issues could lead to relapse.

  - Encourage family members to attend Al-Anon, a support group for relatives of people who misuse alcohol.

Other Substance-Related Disorders

Caffeine-Related Disorders

Caffeine is the most commonly used psychoactive substance in the world. The most potent source of caffeine is coffee, followed by tea and soft drinks. Caffeine also is available in over-the-counter pain and cold remedies. People who use too much caffeine can develop both *caffeine intoxication* and *caffeine withdrawal.*

Mild stimulant effects of caffeine occur at doses of 50–150 mg (i.e., one cup of coffee). Effects include increased alertness and improved verbal and motor performance. At higher dosages, unless tolerance has been achieved, signs of intoxication occur, including restlessness, irritability, and insomnia. Massive doses can lead to seizures and coma. Caffeine withdrawal can cause headaches, lethargy, irritability, and depression.

Because caffeine is well known to aggravate anxiety syndromes such as panic disorder and generalized anxiety disorder, always ask patients about their caffeine intake. Chronic use itself can cause excessive anxiety; in DSM-5, this condition is called *caffeine-induced anxiety disorder.* Caffeine intake can contribute to excess gastric acidity, and thereby worsen esophageal and gastric disorders, and can exacerbate fibrocystic breast disease in women. Caffeine is an underrecognized cause of insomnia.

Once caffeine intoxication is diagnosed, treatment consists of reducing or gradually eliminating caffeine from the diet.

Cannabis-Related Disorders

In DSM-5, cannabis-related disorders include cannabis intoxication, cannabis withdrawal, and cannabis use disorder. *Cannabis* is a general term that also refers to other forms including natural and synthetic cannabinoid compounds. The active ingredient in these formulations is Δ-9-tetrahydrocannabinol (THC), which acts on CB_1 and CB_2 cannabinoid receptors found throughout the central nervous system. About 6% of adults in the United States have a lifetime cannabis use disorder.

Commonly smoked, cannabis sometimes is ingested orally by mixing it into food. Also, devices that vaporize cannabis have been developed. THC and its metabolites are lipid soluble and accumulate in fat cells. The half-life is approximately 50 hours. Intoxication can last 2–4 hours, depending on the dosage, although behavioral changes could continue for many hours.

During *cannabis intoxication*, users could feel a sense of euphoria and serenity. Users develop increased appetite and thirst, feel that their senses are heightened, and report improved self-confidence. Unwanted effects include conjunctivitis, tachycardia, dry mouth, and coughing fits. Psychological effects can include perceptual distortions, sensitivity to sound, and memory impairment. Users also can develop feelings of anxiety and paranoia, impaired attention, and decreased motor coordination. Cannabis use is associated with development of psychotic disorders.

Cannabis withdrawal is characterized by irritability and nervousness, insomnia, poor appetite, restlessness, and depressed mood. Physical signs can include tremors, sweating, fever, chills, and headache.

Benzodiazepines can help calm highly anxious users. There is no specific treatment for withdrawal, but temporary use of a benzodiazepine, a sedative-hypnotic to promote sleep, and nonsteroidal anti-inflammatory drugs can help.

Hallucinogen-Related Disorders

Hallucinogens are a diverse group of compounds, mostly synthetic, that can induce hallucinations, perceptual disturbances, and feelings of unreality. The best known are LSD (lysergic acid diethylamide), mescaline, MDMA (3,4-methylenedioxymethamphetamine), and psilocybin. Phencyclidine (PCP) ("angel dust") is included in the classification because it has hallucinogenic properties.

As sympathomimetics, hallucinogens can cause tachycardia, hypertension, sweating, blurry vision, pupillary dilation, and tremors. They affect several neurotransmitter systems, including dopamine, serotonin, acetylcholine, and γ-aminobutyric acid (GABA) systems. Tolerance to the euphoric and psychedelic effects of hallucinogens develops rapidly.

LSD is short acting and rapidly absorbed. Onset of action occurs within an hour of ingestion, and effects last 6–12 hours. In addition to autonomic hyperarousal, the drug causes profound alterations in perception (e.g., colors may be experienced as brighter and more intense), and senses appear heightened. Emotions seem to intensify, and many users report becoming more introspective. An undesirable outcome is the *flashback*, a brief reexperiencing of the drug's effects that occurs in situations unrelated to taking the drug. In DSM-5, this is diagnosed as *hallucinogen persisting perception disorder*.

Several new "designer" drugs have become popular, including MDMA, better known as "Ecstasy" or "Molly." Mainly used by youth and young adults, it induces an intense feeling of attachment and connection to others and high energy. Other effects include altered time perception, a sense of peacefulness, euphoria, increased desire for sex, and heightened sensory perceptions. The drug also can lead to anxiety, depression, and psychosis.

Hallucinogens do not have a withdrawal syndrome, but benzodiazepines have been used to help calm users who experience an adverse reaction when "talking them down" (i.e., explaining that their reaction is due to the drug and providing reassurance) does not work. Overdose can be a medical emergency. Hyperpyrexia, tachycardia, arrhythmias, stroke, dehydration, or even death can result.

PCP can be administered orally, intravenously, or intranasally. Onset of action occurs in as little as 5 minutes and peaks in about 30 minutes. Users report euphoria, derealization, tingling sensations, and a feeling of warmth. With moderate dosages, bizarre behavior can occur, along with myoclonic jerks, confusion, and disorientation. Higher dosages can produce coma and seizures; death can result from respiratory depression. PCP users have normal or small pupils, unlike hallucinogen users. Chronic psychotic episodes can follow its use. PCP also can cause long-term cognitive deficits. Benzodiazepines can be used to treat agitation, but severe behavioral disturbances may require short-term use of an antipsychotic.

Inhalant-Related Disorders

Inhalants include paint thinner, gasoline, airplane glue, and household cleaners. The active substances are toluene, acetone, benzene, and other organic hydrocarbons. Because inhalants are widely available and cheap, they are used by young persons who have trouble gaining access to other psychoactive substances.

Symptoms include a pattern of use; craving; and impaired social, occupational, or recreational functioning; as well as evidence of tolerance or withdrawal. DSM-5 also recognizes other inhalant substances that may produce inhalant use disorder: nitrous oxide gas, available as a propellant in whipped cream dispensers or diverted from medical or dental sources, and amyl, butyl, and isobutyl nitrate gases, sold as room deodorizers. Inhalants are dangerous because they can damage the CNS, liver, kidneys, and bone marrow. They enter the bloodstream quickly and have rapid onset of action. Inhalants are CNS depressants and produce intoxication similar to that of alcohol but with shorter duration. Effects can last 5–45 minutes and include feelings of excitation, disinhibition, and euphoria. Adverse effects include dizziness, slurred speech, and ataxia. Inhalants also can induce an acute delirium characterized by impaired concentration and disorientation. Hallucinations and delusions have been reported with their use. Other effects include loss of appetite, lateral nystagmus, hypoactive reflexes, and double vision. At higher dosages of inhalant active ingredients, patients could become stuporous or comatose.

There is no specific withdrawal syndrome. Because inhalants often contain high concentrations of heavy metals, permanent neuromuscular and brain damage can occur; kidneys, liver, and other organs are at serious risk of damage from benzene and other hydrocarbons.

Opioid-Related Disorders

Opioids include natural and synthetic substances with morphine-like actions that are full agonists to the mu-opioid receptor. They include morphine, heroin, hydrocodone, oxycodone, codeine, tramadol, and meperidine. Opioids are prescribed as analgesics, anesthetics, antidiarrheal agents, and cough suppressants. Buprenorphine, a drug with both opiate agonist and antagonist effects, is included in this class. Besides heroin, opium is the most widely consumed illegal opiate in the world. Opioid abuse is more common in urban settings, in men, and in ethnic minorities. The course of opioid addiction varies and depends on availability of the drug and exposure. For many, the course is chronic and relapsing.

Opioid users are at high risk for medical conditions resulting from malnutrition and use of dirty needles: hepatitis B and C infection, HIV infection, pneumonia, skin ulcers at injection sites, and cellulitis. Opioid addiction is associated with high mortality rates because of inadvertent fatal overdoses, deaths from accidents ("silent death"), and suicide.

Opioids can be injected, snorted, or smoked, producing euphoria and a sense of well-being. Drowsiness, inactivity, psychomotor retardation, and impaired concentration follow. Physical signs include flushing, pupillary constriction, slurred speech, respiratory depression, hypotension, hypothermia, and bradycardia. Constipation, nausea, and vomiting also are frequent.

Tolerance to most of these drug effects, including the initial euphoria, eventually develops. In chronic users, depending on dosage and drug potency, *withdrawal symptoms* begin approximately 10 hours after the last dose with short-acting opioids (e.g., morphine, heroin) or after a longer period with longer-acting substances (e.g., methadone):

- Minor withdrawal symptoms: lacrimation, rhinorrhea, sweating, yawning, piloerection, hypertension, and tachycardia
- More severe withdrawal symptoms: hot and cold flashes, muscle and joint pain, nausea, vomiting, and abdominal cramps

Clinicians are encouraged to use the Clinical Opiate Withdrawal Scale, or COWS, to assess withdrawal symptoms.

Seizures sometimes occur during meperidine withdrawal. Psychological symptoms of opioid withdrawal include severe anxiety and restlessness, irritability, insomnia, and decreased appetite.

There are two options for treating opioid withdrawal: 1) opioid replacement, and 2) non-opioid treatment for symptomatic relief. Usually methadone or buprenorphine are used to treat opioid withdrawal. A federal "3-day rule" states that opioids should not be given for detoxification for more than 72 hours if the prescriber is not part of a narcotic treatment program. This rule is not intended to obstruct medical care, and an extended detoxification period is allowed if medically necessary. With methadone, clinicians might start with 10–20 mg orally for the first dose and give an additional 5–10 mg if withdrawal symptoms persist after 1 hour. The patient should receive no more than 40 mg in the first day. If the goal is a 3-

day taper, the dosage can then be cut by 50% on days 2 and 3, or if a longer taper is preferred, the dosage can be reduced more slowly. Methadone can be given in two or three divided doses daily. Record the patient's vital signs before each dose.

With buprenorphine, start with a 2- to 4-mg dose when the patient has moderate withdrawal symptoms, and titrate to a maximum of 12–16 mg in the first day in divided doses (taken sublingually). After the patient has stabilized for 2 days, buprenorphine can be tapered over 3–6 days. The taper could be done in 3 days if necessary by reducing the dosage by 50% per day.

Non-opioid withdrawal typically involves the use of clonidine, which suppresses autonomic signs of withdrawal. Clinicians should start with 0.1 mg every 4–6 hours as needed for withdrawal symptoms. The dose can be increased to a maximum of 1.2 mg/day in divided doses. The medication can then be slowly tapered over 7–10 days. Benzodiazepines can be used to treat mild cases of withdrawal and have the advantage of relieving anxiety and promoting needed sleep. Nonsteroidal anti-inflammatory drugs can relieve muscle aches and pain. Gastrointestinal distress can be treated with dicyclomine.

Methadone maintenance requires enrollment in a federally licensed medical clinic; therefore, it cannot be started in the hospital. In these clinics, methadone is administered orally (e.g., 60–100 mg/day). In contrast, buprenorphine maintenance *can* be started in a hospital by any practitioner with a Drug Addiction Treatment Act waiver. The rationale behind replacement therapy is that by switching addicted persons to methadone, drug hunger is alleviated so that the patient is less preoccupied with drug-seeking behavior. People enrolled in these programs have significant decreases in opioid and non-opioid drug use, criminal activity, and depressive symptoms.

Sedative-, Hypnotic-, and Anxiolytic-Related Disorders: Benzodiazepines

Sedative, hypnotic, and anxiolytic substances include benzodiazepines, benzodiazepine-like drugs, carbonates, barbiturates, and barbiturate-like hypnotics. This classification includes all prescription sleeping medications and almost all antianxiety medications. Because barbiturates are prescribed rarely, this section will only involve discussion of the benzodiazepines. About 1 in 20 adults in the United States fill a benzodiazepine prescription during a given year.

Rational Prescribing of Benzodiazepines[1]

1. Avoid or limit prescriptions to patients if risk of substance abuse is suggested by

    - A history of alcohol misuse.

    - A history of drug misuse.

    - The presence of antisocial or borderline personality disorder.

    - A strong family history of substance misuse.

2. Learn to recognize "red flag" presentations in patients seeking prescription drugs, as suggested by

    - Dramatic claims of need for a scheduled drug.

    - Reports of lost prescriptions.

    - Frequent requests for early refills.

    - Requests for a specific scheduled drug, reports of allergies to other drugs, or use of nonscheduled drugs for pain relief or anxiety.

    - Obtaining prescriptions from many physicians ("doctor-shopping").

[1] Courtesy of William R. Yates, M.D.

Intoxication symptoms are dose-related. Lethargy, impaired mental functioning, poor memory, irritability, self-neglect, and emotional disinhibition all can occur. As intoxication progresses, slurred speech, ataxia, and impaired coordination can develop. Individuals could experience anterograde amnesia. Severe intoxication can result in paradoxical agitation. Although benzodiazepines have a high therapeutic index, respiratory depression could be a concern, particularly in those with compromised pulmonary function, or in those who also use other drugs or alcohol. In those cases, the patient will need medical monitoring in a hospital. Flumazenil can reverse the effects of a benzodiazepine overdose.

Withdrawal varies little from drug to drug, although symptoms might be more intense with the shorter-acting drugs (e.g., alprazolam) and more prolonged with the longer-acting ones (e.g., diazepam). The syndromes are similar to those seen with alcohol use disorders.

Abrupt discontinuation of benzodiazepines leads to anxiety, restlessness, and a feeling of apprehension in the first 24 hours. Coarse tremors soon develop, and deep tendon reflexes become hyperactive. Weakness, nausea and vomiting, ortho-static hypotension, sweating, and other signs of autonomic hyperarousal occur. Withdrawal from short-acting benzo-diazepines (e.g., alprazolam) can predispose individuals to seizures.

Withdrawal involves a very slow taper of the drug over days or even weeks. Some patients will need detoxification under medical supervision to forestall development of significant withdrawal symptoms. The patient's usual maintenance dosage, if known, can serve as the starting point. Drugs can be discontinued by 10% each day in the hospital, or 10% every week or two in outpatients. Reevaluate the taper throughout to ensure that the rate is clinically appropriate and safe. The first half of the taper tends to be better tolerated. It might make sense to substitute a long-acting benzodiazepine (e.g., clonaz-epam) for patients who abused a shorter-acting benzodiaze-pine (e.g., alprazolam).

Stimulant-Related Disorders

Stimulants include dextroamphetamine, methylphenidate, methamphetamine, cocaine, and several other substances that share similar pharmacological activity. These substances elevate mood, increase energy and alertness, decrease appetite, and improve task performance. These drugs also cause autonomic hyperarousal, which leads to tachycardia, elevated blood pressure, and pupillary dilation.

The abuse potential of stimulants was recognized relatively early because of their overuse as diet pills. More recently, their abuse has increased along with the rise in diagnosed attention-deficit/hyperactivity disorder, which commonly is treated with stimulants.

Stimulants are also associated with intoxication and with-drawal syndromes. Stimulant intoxication is diagnosed on the basis of recent use, maladaptive behavior, and evidence of autonomic hyperarousal.

Cocaine differs structurally from the amphetamines but has similar effects. Cocaine intoxication could induce tactile hallucinations (e.g., "coke bugs"); in DSM-5, this can be spec-ified as a "perceptual disturbance." Psychological symptoms of cocaine use include a sense of euphoria, disinhibition, sex-ual arousal, enhanced feelings of mastery, and improved self-esteem. Depending on how the drug is administered (e.g., in-tranasally, intravenously), users might experience a rapid onset of euphoria, or "rush." Users smoking a purified cocaine base freed from its salts and cutting agents (i.e., freebasing) report an even more rapid, but short-lived, high.

Stimulant intoxication can induce aggression, agitation, and impaired judgment. A paranoid psychosis similar to that seen in patients with schizophrenia can develop but usually subsides 1–2 weeks after drug use stops. If a stimulant-induced psychosis persists, consider a diagnosis of schizophrenia if it is clear that there is no continuing source of the drug. Delirium is a rare complication that gradually resolves after the drug has been discontinued. Cocaine also has been associated with serious medical complications, such as acute myocardial infarction due to coronary artery constriction and anoxic brain damage due to cocaine-induced seizures.

Cessation or reduction of a stimulant drug can lead to symptoms of withdrawal commonly referred to as a "crash." Symptoms include fatigue and depression, nightmares, headache, profuse sweating, muscle cramps, and hunger. Symptoms usually peak in 2–4 days. Intense dysphoria can occur, peaking 48–72 hours after the last stimulant dose.

Because intoxication and stimulant-induced psychotic disorder generally are self-limiting, no specific treatment is necessary. Benzodiazepines can be used to treat agitation or anxiety. Antipsychotics have been used for stimulant-induced psychoses but usually are unnecessary because the psychosis is short-lived once the drug has been stopped. A withdrawal depression that persists for more than 2 weeks can be treated with antidepressants, although their use in these cases has not been systematically evaluated. No medications have been consistently effective for treating stimulant dependence. Cognitive-behavioral therapy appears promising.

Tobacco-Related Disorders

Approximately 20% of adult Americans smoke, although smoking is more frequent among specific groups (e.g., minority groups, persons with lower income, persons with less education). Rates of smoking among psychiatric patients also are very high. For example, alcohol- or drug-abusing patients are highly likely to smoke, and nearly 90% of patients with schizophrenia smoke.

Nicotine withdrawal usually begins within 1 hour after the last cigarette is smoked and peaks within 24 hours. Withdrawal could last weeks or months and consists of nicotine craving, irritability, anxiety, restlessness, and decreased heart rate. Weight gain and depression often follow smoking cessation.

There are several FDA-approved treatments for smoking cessation, including nicotine transdermal patches and nicotine-containing gum, lozenges, and inhalers; bupropion; and varenicline (Chantix). The combination of nicotine-replacement patches or gum with bupropion or varenicline could work even better.

Other Specified Substance-Related and Addictive Disorders

- *Anabolic steroids* are widely abused by athletes who believe that the drugs will enhance their performance and muscle mass. Although these drugs initially may produce a sense of well-being, this feeling is later replaced by anergy, dysphoria, and irritability. Frank psychosis can develop, as can serious medical problems, including liver disease.
- *Nitrate inhalants* ("poppers") produce an intoxicated state characterized by a feeling of fullness in the head, mild euphoria, a change in time perception, relaxation of the smooth muscles, and possibly an increase in sexual feelings. These drugs carry the possible risk of immune system impairment, respiratory system irritation, and a toxic reaction that could lead to vomiting, severe headaches, and hypotension.
- *Nitrous oxide* ("laughing gas") can cause intoxication characterized by light-headedness and a floating sensation that quickly clears once administration of the gas stops. Temporary confusion or paranoia can result when this substance is used regularly.

Clinical Points for Substance-Related Disorders

- Do not allow your personal beliefs and attitudes about drug use to interfere with care of the addicted patient.
  - Patients need a consistent yet firm approach.
  - Neither condemn addicted persons nor condone their behavior.

- Assess the patient for medical and psychiatric comorbidity. Many substance-abusing persons have potentially serious medical problems that require treatment, significant use of other substances, co-occurring mood and anxiety disorders, or a personality disorder.

- Be prepared for relapses during the continuation phase of treatment. Relapse is nearly inevitable, but it does not represent failure of the treatment program. The clinician must be there to help the patient get back on the wagon.

- Support groups can be very helpful to the patient, and referral to community-based organizations is essential.

Non-Substance-Related Disorders: Gambling Disorder

Gambling disorder, formerly *pathological gambling*, was moved to the addictions chapter because of research showing its close connection to substance-related disorders. The DSM-5 criteria for gambling disorder are listed in Box 15–2.

Box 15–2. DSM-5 Criteria for Gambling Disorder

A. Persistent and recurrent problematic gambling behavior leading to clinically significant impairment or distress, as indicated by the individual exhibiting four (or more) of the following in a 12-month period:

1. Needs to gamble with increasing amounts of money in order to achieve the desired excitement.
2. Is restless or irritable when attempting to cut down or stop gambling.
3. Has made repeated unsuccessful efforts to control, cut back, or stop gambling.
4. Is often preoccupied with gambling (e.g., having persistent thoughts of reliving past gambling experiences, handicapping or planning the next venture, thinking of ways to get money with which to gamble).
5. Often gambles when feeling distressed (e.g., helpless, guilty, anxious, depressed).

6. After losing money gambling, often returns another day to get even ("chasing" one's losses).
7. Lies to conceal the extent of involvement with gambling.
8. Has jeopardized or lost a significant relationship, job, or educational or career opportunity because of gambling.
9. Relies on others to provide money to relieve desperate financial situations caused by gambling.

B. The gambling behavior is not better explained by a manic episode.

Gambling disorder affects 0.4%–2% of the general population. Two-thirds of people with gambling disorder are male. Women take up gambling later than men but tend to develop gambling disorder more quickly. Mood and anxiety disorders, substance use disorders, and personality disorders often are comorbid. Gambling disorder runs in families and appears genetically related to substance use disorders and antisocial personality disorder.

The opioid antagonists naltrexone and nalmefene (unavailable in the United States) have been shown to reduce gambling urges. The selective serotonin reuptake inhibitors might be helpful, particularly in depressed or anxious persons with gambling disorder. Referral to Gamblers Anonymous, a 12-step program similar to Alcoholics Anonymous, could be helpful. Cognitive-behavioral therapy can address the irrational thoughts and beliefs associated with gambling. Motivational interviewing can encourage patients to make needed changes in their behavior.

Further Reading

American Psychiatric Association: Practice guideline for the treatment of patients with substance use disorders, second edition. Am J Psychiatry 164 (4, suppl):5–123, 2007

Anton RF, O'Malley SS, Ciraulo DA, et al; COMBINE Study Research Group: Combined pharmacotherapies and behavioral interventions for alcohol dependence: the COMBINE study: a randomized controlled trial. JAMA 295(17):2003–2017, 2006

Compton WM, Dawson DA, Conway KP, et al: Transitions in illicit drug use status over 3 years: a prospective analysis of a general population sample. Am J Psychiatry 170(6):660–670, 2013

Ewing JA: Detecting alcoholism. The CAGE questionnaire. JAMA 252(14):1905–1907, 1984

Galanter M, Kleber HD, Brady KT (eds): The American Psychiatric Publishing Textbook of Substance Abuse Treatment, 5th Edition. Washington, DC, American Psychiatric Publishing, 2015

Goldstein RZ, Volkow ND: Dysfunction of the prefrontal cortex in addiction: neuroimaging findings and clinical implications. Nat Rev Neurosci 12(11):652–669, 2011

Grant BF, Goldstein RB, Saha TD, et al: Epidemiology of DSM-5 Alcohol Use Disorder: results from the National Epidemiologic Survey on Alcohol and Related Conditions III. JAMA Psychiatry 72(8):757–766, 2015

Grant JE, Potenza MN, Hollander E, et al: Multicenter investigation of the opioid antagonist nalmefene in the treatment of pathological gambling. Am J Psychiatry 163(2):303–312, 2006

Hasin DS, Kerridge BT, Saha TD, et al: Prevalence and correlates of DSM-5 cannabis use disorder, 2012-2013: findings from the National Epidemiologic Survey of Alcohol and Related Conditions-III. Am J Psychiatry 173(6):588–599, 2016

Howard MO, Bowen SE, Garland EL, et al: Inhalant use and inhalant use disorders in the United States. Addict Sci Clin Pract 6(1):18–31, 2011

Kalivas PW, Volkow ND: The neural basis of addiction: a pathology of motivation and choice. Am J Psychiatry 162(8):1403–1413, 2005

Levounis P, Zerbo E, Aggarwal R: Pocket Guide to Addiction Assessment and Treatment. Arlington, VA, American Psychiatric Association Publishing, 2016

Olfson M, King M, Schoenbaum M: Benzodiazepine use in the United States. JAMA Psychiatry 72(2):136–142, 2015

Satre DD, Chi FW, Mertens JR, Weisner CM: Effects of age and life transitions on alcohol and drug treatment outcome over nine years. J Stud Alcohol Drugs 73(3):459–468, 2012

Schuckit MA: Alcohol-use disorders. Lancet 373(9662):492–501, 2009

Chapter 16

Neurocognitive Disorders

Neurocognitive disorders involve structural or functional disturbances of brain function leading to impairments in memory, abstract thinking, or judgment. They are acquired rather than developmental and are associated with a clinically significant decline in a person's level of functioning. The DSM-5 neurocognitive disorders are listed in Table 16–1.

DSM-5 has introduced two new categories—*major neurocognitive disorder* and *mild neurocognitive disorder*—that are distinguished on the basis of severity. The term *dementia* has been replaced with *neurocognitive disorder*, although the former often is used to describe the etiological subtypes. The criteria for major and mild neurocognitive disorder are based on six key cognitive domains:

- *Complex attention:* sustained attention, divided attention, selective attention, processing speed
- *Executive function:* planning, decision making, working memory, responding to feedback/error correction, overriding habits, mental flexibility
- *Learning and memory:* immediate memory, recent memory (including free recall, cued recall, and recognition memory)
- *Language:* expressive language (including naming, fluency, and grammar and syntax) and receptive language
- *Perceptual motor ability:* construction and visual perception
- *Social cognition:* recognition of emotions, theory of mind (i.e., ability to understand another person's mental state), behavioral regulation

Delirium

The hallmark of delirium is rapid development of disorientation, confusion, and global cognitive impairment that can fluctuate during the course of a day. Delirium is the result of the direct physiological consequences of a medical condition, substance intoxication or withdrawal, exposure to a toxin, or

TABLE 16–1. DSM-5 neurocognitive disorders

Delirium

  Other specified delirium

  Unspecified delirium

Major neurocognitive disorder

Mild neurocognitive disorder

Subtypes of major or mild neurocognitive disorder

  Due to Alzheimer's disease

  Frontotemporal neurocognitive disorder

  With Lewy bodies

  Vascular neurocognitive disorder

  Due to traumatic brain injury

  Substance/medication-induced

  Due to HIV infection

  Due to prion disease

  Due to Parkinson's disease

  Due to Huntington's disease

  Due to another medical condition

  Due to multiple etiologies

multiple etiologies. The DSM-5 criteria for delirium are shown in Box 16–1.

Box 16–1. DSM-5 Criteria for Delirium

A. A disturbance in attention (i.e., reduced ability to direct, focus, sustain, and shift attention) and awareness (reduced orientation to the environment).

B. The disturbance develops over a short period of time (usually hours to a few days), represents a change from baseline attention and awareness, and tends to fluctuate in severity during the course of a day.

C. An additional disturbance in cognition (e.g., memory deficit, disorientation, language, visuospatial ability, or perception).

D. The disturbances in Criteria A and C are not better explained by another preexisting, established, or evolving neurocognitive disorder and do not occur in the context of a severely reduced level of arousal, such as coma.

E. There is evidence from the history, physical examination, or laboratory findings that the disturbance is a direct physiological consequence of another medical condition, substance intoxication or withdrawal (i.e., due to a drug of abuse or to a medication), or exposure to a toxin, or is due to multiple etiologies.

Delirium affects an estimated 10%–15% of medical patients and is common in hospitals. Elderly patients, especially those older than 80 years, are at high risk. Other risk factors include preexisting dementia, recent surgery, bone fractures, systemic infections, and recent use of narcotics or antipsychotics. Approximately 40%–50% of patients with delirium die within 1 year.

Clinical Findings

Typical features include reduced clarity of awareness of the environment; difficulty focusing, sustaining, or shifting attention; impaired cognition; and perceptual disturbances (e.g., illusions). Other symptoms include sleep-wake cycle disturbances that worsen at night ("sundowning"); disorientation to place, date, or person; incoherence; restlessness; agitation; and excessive somnolence.

Etiology

Because delirium is a *syndrome*, not a disease, it is best considered the final common pathway of many potential causes that include metabolic disturbances from infection, febrile illness, hypoxia, hypoglycemia, drug intoxication or withdrawal states, or hepatic encephalopathy. Potential causes that lie *within* the central nervous system (CNS) include brain abscesses, stroke, traumatic injuries, and postictal states. Other potential causes include new-onset arrhythmias (e.g., atrial fibrillation) and cardiac ischemia.

Assessment

Evaluation begins with a detailed history and physical examination. Interview informants because the patient probably will not be able to provide a history. Pay close attention to the presence of focal neurological signs, such as weakness/

sensory loss or papilledema. Frontal lobe release signs (e.g., suck, snout, palmomental, rooting reflexes), if present, could indicate global brain dysfunction.

The medical workup should include routine blood and urine studies (e.g., complete blood count, urinalysis), chest radiography, a brain computed tomography (CT) or magnetic resonance imaging (MRI) scan, an electrocardiogram, lumbar puncture (in selected patients), toxicology screen, blood gases, and an electroencephalogram (EEG).

Serum urine toxicology is essential for patients presenting to emergency departments to evaluate for illicit drug use. Delirious patients frequently have temperature elevations that likely represent autonomic instability or an underlying infection. Generalized diffuse slowing often is found on the EEG.

Clinical Management

The underlying medical condition, if known, must be corrected. Measures to maintain the patient's health and safety include constant observation, consistent nursing care, and frequent reassurance with repeated simple explanations. Minimize external stimulation. Delirious patients tend to do better in quiet, well-lit rooms.

Discontinue unnecessary medication, including sedative-hypnotics (e.g., benzodiazepines). Not only are delirious patients sensitive to drug adverse effects, but the drugs could contribute to the delirium. Agitated patients could be calmed with low dosages of high-potency antipsychotics (e.g., haloperidol, 1–2 mg every 2–4 hours as needed) or a low dosage of a second-generation antipsychotic (SGA). Avoid medications with significant anticholinergic activity (e.g., chlorpromazine) because they can worsen or prolong the delirium.

If sedation is necessary, low dosages of short-acting benzodiazepines (e.g., oxazepam, lorazepam) can be helpful. Unrecognized alcohol withdrawal can manifest as delirium, particularly in postsurgical patients who did not report a history of alcohol misuse. In these cases, benzodiazepines can be helpful.

Clinical Points for Delirium

- In the hospital, ensure that the confused patient has a quiet, restful setting that is well lighted.

- Maintain consistency of personnel, which is less likely to upset the delirious patient.

- Prominently display reminders of day, date, time, place, and situation in the patient's room.

- Limit medication for behavioral management to patients who did not respond to behavioral interventions.

  - Prescribe only essential drugs and avoid polypharmacy.

  - Avoid sedatives, hypnotics, and anxiolytics; the exception is when the delirium is due to alcohol withdrawal.

  - Unmanageable behavior might require the use of high-potency antipsychotics (e.g., haloperidol) or, alternatively, benzodiazepines with short half-lives (e.g., lorazepam).

Major and Mild Neurocognitive Disorders

Level of impairment distinguishes major and mild neurocognitive disorder. *Major neurocognitive disorder* causes "significant" cognitive decline and "substantial" impairment in cognitive performance; in addition, deficits "interfere" with independence in everyday living. With *mild neurocognitive disorder*, cognitive decline and impairment in cognitive function are "modest," and the deficits do not interfere with capacity for independence in everyday activities. The DSM-5 criteria for major neurocognitive disorder are presented in Box 16–2. Because the criteria for mild neurocognitive disorder are similar—except for the distinctions noted—they are not reproduced here.

Box 16–2.   DSM-5 Criteria for Major
                    Neurocognitive Disorder

A. Evidence of significant cognitive decline from a previous level of performance in one or more cognitive domains (complex attention, executive function, learning and memory, language, perceptual-motor, or social cognition) based on:

  1. Concern of the individual, a knowledgeable informant, or the clinician that there has been a significant decline in cognitive function; and

2. A substantial impairment in cognitive performance, preferably documented by standardized neuropsychological testing or, in its absence, another quantified clinical assessment.

B. The cognitive deficits interfere with independence in everyday activities (i.e., at a minimum, requiring assistance with complex instrumental activities of daily living such as paying bills or managing medications).

C. The cognitive deficits do not occur exclusively in the context of a delirium.

D. The cognitive deficits are not better explained by another mental disorder (e.g., major depressive disorder, schizophrenia).

Specify whether due to:
Alzheimer's disease
Frontotemporal lobar degeneration
Lewy body disease
Vascular disease
Traumatic brain injury
Substance/medication use
HIV infection
Prion disease
Parkinson's disease
Huntington's disease
Another medical condition
Multiple etiologies
Unspecified

The core feature of major and mild neurocognitive disorder is a decline in one or more cognitive domains based on the following:

- The patient's history (reported by the patient and/or knowledgeable informants), and
- Performance on an objective assessment that falls below expectation or has declined over time.

Major neurocognitive disorders are uncommon among people younger than 65 years. The percentage of those affected is linear. Among those ages 65–75, about 10% will be affected; at age 90 approximately 50% will be affected. The rates of major neurocognitive disorder are even higher among elderly hospitalized patients and physically ill persons.

Clinical Findings

Other than abrupt-onset disorders (e.g., strokes), most neurocognitive disorders develop insidiously. Early signs could be overlooked or misattributed to normal aging. Early on, the only symptom could be a subtle change in the person's personality, a decrease in the range of the person's interests, or the development of apathy. Intellectual skills are affected gradually and might be noticed initially in work settings that require high performance.

Cognitive impairment becomes more pronounced as the disorder advances. Mood and personality changes become exaggerated, and psychotic symptoms can develop. When the disorder is in an advanced stage, the patient may not be able to perform basic tasks such as self-feeding or personal hygiene. Patients frequently forget names of friends and sometimes are unable to recognize close relatives. In its end stage, a patient may be mute and unresponsive.

Temper outbursts, wandering, paranoia, and poor hygiene are often the most troublesome symptoms from the family member's viewpoint. Approximately one-half of patients with Alzheimer's disease develop hallucinations and/or delusions. Nearly 20% of Alzheimer's disease patients also develop major depression, and perhaps an equal number will have milder depressive symptoms. Depression is even more common among patients with vascular forms of neurocognitive disorder.

Diagnosis and Assessment

The history, physical examination, and mental status examination are the best tools to detect neurocognitive disorders. Two "bedside" tests are available to assess the person's orientation, memory, constructional ability, and the ability to read, write, and calculate:

- Mini-Mental State Examination (MMSE)
- Montreal Cognitive Assessment (MoCA)

A medical workup will help rule out treatable causes of the neurocognitive disorder, although most are irreversible (Table 16–2). Other laboratory tests are helpful in select patients. A CT or an MRI brain scan is appropriate in the presence of a history that suggests a mass lesion, focal neurological signs, or a rapid onset of neurocognitive disorder. EEGs are appropriate for patients with altered consciousness or suspected seizures. Pulse oximetry is indicated when compromised pul-

TABLE 16–2. Medical workup for neurocognitive disorders

1. Complete history

2. Thorough physical examination, including neurological examination

3. Mental status examination

4. Laboratory studies

   - Complete blood count, with differential
   - Serum electrolytes
   - Serum glucose
   - Blood urea nitrogen
   - Creatinine
   - Liver function tests
   - Serology for syphilis and HIV
   - Thyroid function tests
   - Serum vitamin B_{12}
   - Folate
   - Urinalysis and urine drug screen
   - Electrocardiogram
   - Chest X-ray
   - Pulse oximetry
   - Brain computed tomography or magnetic resonance imaging

5. Neuropsychological testing (e.g., attention, memory, cognitive function)

6. Optional tests

   - Functional neuroimaging (e.g., positron emission tomography, single-photon emission computed tomography)
   - Lumbar puncture

monary function is evident. Single-photon emission computed tomography (SPECT) or positron emission tomography (PET) can help distinguish Alzheimer's disease from other forms of neurocognitive disorder. In Alzheimer's disease, patients show characteristic temporal and parietal hypometabolism.

TABLE 16–3. Clinical features differentiating dementia and delirium

Dementia	Delirium
Chronic or insidious	Acute onset
Sensorium unimpaired early on	Sensorium clouded
Normal level of arousal	Agitation or stupor
Progressive and deteriorating	Often reversible
Common in nursing homes and psychiatric hospitals	Common on medical, surgical, and neurological wards

Neuropsychological testing can be helpful as part of the overall evaluation of the patient. Testing can be done to

- Obtain baseline data to measure change before and after treatment.
- Evaluate highly educated individuals suspected of developing early dementia when brain imaging or other test results are ambiguous.
- Help distinguish delirium from dementia and depression. Serially track changes in attention, memory, and cognition.

Because symptoms of dementia and delirium overlap, it is important to separate the syndromes (Table 16–3).

It is equally important to separate major neurocognitive disorder from the *dementia syndrome of depression* (pseudodementia): the depressed patient might not be able to remember correctly, cannot calculate well, and complains of lost cognitive abilities. The importance of this distinction is obvious: a patient with pseudodementia has a treatable illness (depression) and does not have dementia.

Etiological Subtypes of Major or Mild Neurocognitive Disorder

Alzheimer's Disease

Alzheimer's disease is the most common form of major neurocognitive disorder, accounting for 50%–60% of cases and affecting approximately 2.5 million Americans. In DSM-5,

Alzheimer's disease is divided into probable and possible types. With *probable* Alzheimer's disease, there is evidence of either 1) a causative genetic mutation from family history or genetic testing or 2) decline in memory and learning and at least one other cognitive domain; steadily progressive decline; and no evidence of mixed etiology. If neither is present, possible Alzheimer's disease is diagnosed. The DSM-5 criteria for major or mild neurocognitive disorder due to Alzheimer's disease are shown in Box 16–3.

Box 16–3. DSM-5 Criteria for Major or Mild Neurocognitive Disorder Due to Alzheimer's Disease

---

A. The criteria are met for major or mild neurocognitive disorder.

B. There is insidious onset and gradual progression of impairment in one or more cognitive domains (for major neurocognitive disorder, at least two domains must be impaired).

C. Criteria are met for either probable or possible Alzheimer's disease as follows:

For major neurocognitive disorder:

Probable Alzheimer's disease is diagnosed if either of the following is present; otherwise, **possible Alzheimer's disease** should be diagnosed.

1. Evidence of a causative Alzheimer's disease genetic mutation from family history or genetic testing.

2. All three of the following are present:

   a. Clear evidence of decline in memory and learning and at least one other cognitive domain (based on detailed history or serial neuropsychological testing).

   b. Steadily progressive, gradual decline in cognition, without extended plateaus.

   c. No evidence of mixed etiology (i.e., absence of other neurodegenerative or cerebrovascular disease, or another neurological, mental, or systemic disease or condition likely contributing to cognitive decline).

For mild neurocognitive disorder:

Probable Alzheimer's disease is diagnosed if there is evidence of a causative Alzheimer's disease genetic mutation from either genetic testing or family history.

Possible Alzheimer's disease is diagnosed if there is no evidence of a causative Alzheimer's disease genetic mutation from either genetic testing or family history, and all three of the following are present:

1. Clear evidence of decline in memory and learning.
2. Steadily progressive, gradual decline in cognition, without extended plateaus.
3. No evidence of mixed etiology (i.e., absence of other neurodegenerative or cerebrovascular disease, or another neurological or systemic disease or condition likely contributing to cognitive decline).

D. The disturbance is not better explained by cerebrovascular disease, another neurodegenerative disease, the effects of a substance, or another mental, neurological, or systemic disorder.

Alzheimer's disease usually has an insidious onset leading to death 8–10 years after symptoms are first recognized. Estimates of its prevalence range from 5% at age 65 to 40% by age 90. Symptoms worsen progressively, eventually resulting in near collapse of cognitive functioning. Physical findings, such as hyperactive deep tendon reflexes, Babinski's sign, and frontal lobe release signs, generally are absent or are present only in later stages. Illusions, hallucinations, or delusions are associated with accelerated cognitive deterioration. Cortical atrophy and enlarged cerebral ventricles are typically seen on CT or MRI scans.

Early-onset (age <65 years) patients often have an onset in the fifth decade, and the disorder has been linked to mutations on chromosomes 1, 14, and 21. Most cases are of late onset (≥65 years).

Two primary abnormalities characterize the histopathology of Alzheimer's disease:

- Amyloid plaques that result from an overabundance of β-amyloid 42, a peptide derived from amyloid precursor protein
- Neurofibrillary tangles that are composed of hyperphosphorylated tau protein that folds within the intracellular cytoplasm of neurons

Neurofibrillary tangles also are seen in a variety of neurodegenerative diseases, such as frontotemporal dementia, and in persons with closed head injuries.

Alzheimer's disease risk factors include a history of head injury, Down syndrome, low educational and occupational achievement, and having a first-degree relative with the disorder. Up to 50% of first-degree relatives of persons with Alzheimer's disease develop the disorder by age 90. A genetic polymorphism on chromosome 19, apolipoprotein E (*APOE*), has been found to influence the risk of Alzheimer's disease. The *APOE* ε4 allele increases risk and decreases age at onset, and the *APOE* ε2 allele has a protective effect.

Frontotemporal

Frontotemporal neurocognitive disorder (formerly Pick's disease) accounts for approximately 5% of all cases of dementia and is a relatively common cause of dementia in persons younger than 65 years. There are a behavioral variant and three language variants that have distinct patterns of brain atrophy and some distinctive neuropathology. The *behavioral-variant* subtype presents with varying degrees of apathy or disinhibition. Individuals with the *language-variant* subtype present with primary progressive aphasia of gradual onset. In general, this disorder is characterized by tau-positive inclusions. In a subgroup of patients with frontotemporal neurocognitive disorder—those with parkinsonian features—the disease is linked to a gene on chromosome 17. The disease is progressive, with a median survival of 6–11 years after symptom onset and 3–4 years after diagnosis.

Lewy Bodies

Neurocognitive disorder with Lewy bodies could account for up to 25% of dementia cases and is progressive. In addition to changes in the brain parenchyma typical for Alzheimer's disease, Lewy bodies—eosinophilic inclusion bodies—are present in the cerebral cortex and brainstem. The disorder causes progressive cognitive impairment with early changes in complex attention and executive function rather than learning and memory. Visual and other types of hallucinations, depression, delusions, and signs of autonomic dysfunction (e.g., orthostatic hypotension) can occur. Patients might experience a concurrent rapid eye movement sleep behavior disorder. Another core feature is spontaneous parkinsonism that begins after onset of cognitive decline. A diagnostically suggestive feature is low striatal dopamine transporter uptake on SPECT or PET scans. Up to 50% of individuals with this disorder are highly sensitive to antipsychotic drugs, which should be avoided.

Vascular

Vascular neurocognitive disorder is the second most common cause of dementia after Alzheimer's disease, accounting for 15%–30% of dementia cases; in many patients, the two forms are combined. The diagnosis requires the presence of a dementia and evidence that cerebrovascular disease accounts for the cognitive deficits. Vascular etiology could range from large-vessel stroke to microvascular disease. For that reason, the presentation is heterogeneous because of many types of vascular lesions and their extent and location.

Dementia caused by multiple infarcts probably accounts for most cases and results from accumulation of cerebral infarcts in persons with atherosclerotic disease. Focal neurological deficits (e.g., hemiparesis, visual field deficits) often are present. Lesions can be focal, multifocal, or diffuse and occur in various combinations. Common symptoms are personality and mood changes, loss of motivation, depression, and emotional lability. A history of rapid onset and a stepwise deterioration occurring in patients in their 50s or 60s help distinguish vascular from degenerative forms of dementia.

There is no specific treatment for most forms of the disorder, but as a preventive measure, aim to control blood pressure in those with hypertension and administer anticoagulants or aspirin to help prevent thrombus formation.

Traumatic Brain Injury

Traumatic brain injury is caused by an impact to the head or by other events that cause rapid movement or displacement of the brain within the skull (e.g., improvised explosive devices, or IEDs). Traumatic brain injuries are relatively common, and an estimated 2% of the general population live with such injuries. Symptoms can include initial loss of consciousness, posttraumatic amnesia, disorientation/confusion, or—in more severe cases—neurological signs (e.g., positive neuroimaging, new-onset seizure disorder). To be attributed to traumatic brain injury, the neurocognitive disorder must manifest immediately after the brain injury or immediately after the individual recovers consciousness and must persist past the acute postinjury period.

Traumatic brain injuries can be accompanied by the following:

- Emotional symptoms (e.g., irritability, easy frustration, tension/anxiety, affective lability)
- Personality change (e.g., disinhibition, apathy, suspiciousness, aggression)
- Physical symptoms (e.g., headache, fatigue, sleep disorders, vertigo or dizziness, tinnitus/hyperacusis, photosensitivity, anosmia)

If there is a brain contusion, intracranial hemorrhage, or penetrating injury, a patient might experience additional neurocognitive deficits, such as aphasia, neglect, and constructional dyspraxia.

Substance/Medication-Induced

Major or mild neurocognitive disorder due to substance/medication use should be distinguished from the cognitive impairments commonly seen with substance intoxication or withdrawal. The impairments seen in intoxication or withdrawal usually are reversible, whereas substance/medication-induced neurocognitive disorder is a persisting condition.

Although nonspecific deficits in a range of cognitive abilities can occur with nearly any substance of abuse and many medications, some patterns occur more frequently than others. For example, a neurocognitive disorder due to sedative, hypnotic, or anxiolytic drugs (e.g., benzodiazepines, barbiturates) could show greater disturbances in memory than in other cognitive functions. Neurocognitive disorder induced by alcohol frequently manifests with a combination of impairments in executive-function and memory and learning domains. With alcohol, the neurocognitive disorder usually is mild, except in cases of *Wernicke's encephalopathy*, a clinical syndrome characterized by ophthalmoplegia, ataxic gait, nystagmus, and mental confusion caused by thiamine deficiency associated with chronic alcohol misuse.

HIV Infection

An estimated 25% of individuals with HIV will have signs and symptoms that meet criteria for mild neurocognitive disorder; less than 5% have signs and symptoms that meet criteria for major neurocognitive disorder. HIV-related neurocognitive disorders could result from direct HIV infection of the CNS, intracranial tumors, or infections (e.g., toxoplasmosis, cryptococcosis), or from the indirect effects of systemic disease (e.g., septicemia, hypoxia, electrolyte imbalance). Because neuro-cognitive disorders can occur during the early stages of HIV infection, evaluation for HIV seropositivity is indicated for persons at high risk for infection (e.g., gay men, persons addicted to drugs) who develop otherwise unexplained cognitive, mood, or behavior changes.

Prion Disease

Neurocognitive disorders due to prion disease include those resulting from a group of subacute spongiform encephalopathies such as Creutzfeldt- Jakob disease, variant Creutzfeldt-Jakob disease, kuru, Gerstmann-Sträussler-Scheinker syndrome, and fatal insomnia. They are caused by small proteinaceous particles called *prions*, once called "slow viruses." *Creutzfeldt-Jakob disease* is the best-known prion disease and can be inherited or transmitted (e.g., intracerebral electrodes, grafts of dura mater, corneal transplants). It is a rare, untreatable, rapidly fatal condition. Histopathology shows spongiform changes consisting of fine vacuolation of the neuropil of the gray matter, associated with astrocytosis and neuronal loss.

Parkinson's Disease

Up to 75% of individuals with Parkinson's disease develop dementia during the course of their disease. People with Parkinson's disease who are older and have more severe disease appear more likely to develop cognitive impairment. Features include apathy, depressed mood, anxious mood, hallucinations, delusions, personality changes, rapid eye movement sleep behavior disorder, and excessive daytime sleepiness. Mild neurocognitive disorder often develops relatively early in the course of Parkinson's disease; major impairment typically occurs late. Pimavanserin (Nuplazid) is FDA-approved to treat psychotic features associated with Parkinson's disease.

Huntington's Disease

Huntington's disease is a neuropsychiatric disorder with autosomal-dominant inheritance. Genetic testing shows a CAG trinucleotide repeat expansion in the huntingtin gene (*HTT*), located on chromosome 4. Progressive cognitive impairment is a core feature, with early changes in executive function (i.e., processing speed, organization, and planning) rather than learning and memory. Cognitive and associated behavioral changes often precede the emergence of the typical motor abnormalities of bradykinesia and choreiform movements. The average age at diagnosis is around 40 years. Age at onset is inversely correlated with CAG expansion length. Juvenile Huntington's disease (onset age<20 years) could present more often with bradykinesia, dystonia, and rigidity than with choreiform movements. The disease is progressive and inevitably fatal.

Another Medical Condition

- *Subdural hematomas* are large blood clots caused by disruption of the veins that bridge brain parenchyma and meninges, and they usually result from blunt trauma. Treatment involves surgical evacuation of the clot through a burr hole in the skull.
- *Normal-pressure hydrocephalus* is caused by excessive accumulation of cerebrospinal fluid that gradually dilates the ventricles of the brain in the presence of normal cerebrospinal fluid pressure resulting in the triad of dementia, gait disturbance, and urinary incontinence. Placing a shunt to remove excess fluid can help some patients.
- *Various medical disorders* can cause dementia. Included are chronic infectious processes caused by bacteria (e.g., Whipple's disease), fungi (e.g., cryptococcal infection), or other microorganisms (e.g., syphilis); metabolic diseases of the thyroid, parathyroid, adrenal, and pituitary glands; pulmonary diseases; chronic or acute renal failure and liver failure (i.e., hepatic encephalopathy); and diabetes.
- *Nutritional disorders* can cause or contribute to dementia. Included are pernicious anemia (B_{12} deficiency), folate deficiency, and pellagra (niacin deficiency).
- *Other rare causes* of dementia include diseases of the cerebellum (cerebellar, spinocerebellar, and olivopontocerebellar degeneration), and motor neurons (amyotrophic lateral sclerosis); herpes simplex encephalitis; multiple sclerosis; Wilson's disease (hepatolenticular degeneration); metachromatic leukodystrophy; the adrenoleukodystrophies; and the neuronal storage diseases (e.g., Tay-Sachs disease).

Clinical Management of Major and Mild Neurocognitive Disorders

Five medications are FDA-approved to treat Alzheimer's disease. Four are cholinesterase inhibitors (donepezil, rivastigmine, galantamine, tacrine), which are equally effective and

TABLE 16–4. Cognitive enhancement medications

Drug	Trade name	Dosage range (mg/day)
Donepezil	Aricept	5–10
Galantamine	Reminyl	8–24
Memantine	Namenda	10–20
Rivastigmine	Exelon	1.5–6
Tacrine	Cognex	40–160

slow the rate of cognitive decline. Memantine also is a cognitive enhancer and blocks the *N*-methyl-D-aspartate (NMDA) receptor, one of two receptors that normally binds glutamate. There is a marked variation in response—some patients show tremendous improvement, whereas others show very little improvement. These drugs do not alter the course of the disease and are most effective in persons in the earliest stages of the disease. (See Table 16–4 for a list of the cognitive enhancers.)

Vitamin E (2,000 IU/day) may slow functional decline in people with mild to moderate Alzheimer's disease.

Other medications are used for symptomatic treatment of associated anxiety, psychosis, or depression, including the anxiolytics, antipsychotics, and antidepressants, respectively. Use the lowest effective dosage, because patients with dementia often poorly tolerate drug adverse effects.

Behavioral problems such as irritability, hostility, and aggression are the most difficult problems to manage in patients with dementia. SGAs often are prescribed for behavioral problems in these patients and are moderately effective, but the dosage of these medications needs to be carefully titrated. Warnings by the FDA have emphasized the importance of careful monitoring of SGAs because of an increased mortality risk associated with their use in elderly patients with dementia. Avoid low-potency antipsychotics (e.g., chlorpromazine), because their anticholinergic activity can worsen confusion. The selective serotonin reuptake inhibitor (SSRI) citalopram has been shown to reduce aggression, anxiety, and delusions and is well tolerated. Trazodone, given at bedtime (25–100 mg), can help relieve nighttime agitation or sundowning. Avoid benzodiazepines except for their occasional use in treating acute agitation.

Behavioral strategies can be helpful. A regular and predictable daily schedule, structured activities, and avoiding alcohol, caffeine, and diuretics are important. *Reminiscence group therapy* could help patients maintain their social skills and improve mood and morale.

Clinical Points for Major and Mild Neurocognitive Disorders

- Both at home and in long-term care facilities, patients usually respond better to low-stimulus environments than to high-stimulus situations.

  - Patients with dementia have difficulty interpreting sensory input and easily become overwhelmed.

- Consistency and routine are important for reducing confusion and agitation.

- Families often are overwhelmed by caring for their cognitively impaired relative. The clinician should:

  - Recommend that family members attend support groups (available in most communities).

  - Recommend appropriate reading material.

  - Counsel relatives to minimize confrontational or critical comments.

- Families will need psychological support if the patient requires institutionalization, to lessen the guilt they almost inevitably feel.

- Cognitive enhancers could slow the rate of cognitive decline but will not reverse it. Accompanying depression generally responds to antidepressants, and acute agitation or psychosis could respond to an antipsychotic.

  - SSRIs may be effective in treating agitation, as well as depression and anxiety.

  - Low-potency antipsychotics such as chlorpromazine should be avoided because their anticholinergic activity can worsen confusion.

- High-potency conventional antipsychotics generally are safe (e.g., haloperidol) but can cause pseudoparkinsonism.

- Second-generation antipsychotics could increase mortality risk and should be used with care.

- Trazodone given at bedtime could help relieve nighttime agitation.

Further Reading

American Psychiatric Association: Practice guideline for the treatment of patients with Alzheimer's disease and other dementias, second edition. Am J Psychiatry 164 (12, suppl):5–56, 2007

Blazer DG, Stefens DC (eds): Essentials of Geriatric Psychiatry, 2nd Edition. Washington, DC, American Psychiatric Publishing, 2012

Dysken MW, Sano M, Asthana S, et al: Effect of vitamin E and memantine on functional decline in Alzheimer disease: the TEAM-AD VA cooperative randomized trial. JAMA 311(1):33–44, 2014

Folstein MF, Folstein SE, McHugh PR: "Mini-mental state". A practical method for grading the cognitive state of patients for the clinician. J Psychiatr Res 12(3):189–198, 1975

Howard R, McShane R, Lindesay J, et al: Donepezil and memantine for moderate-to-severe Alzheimer's disease. N Engl J Med 366(10):893–903, 2012

Leonpacher AK, Peters ME, Drye LT, et al; CitAD Research Group: Effects of citalopram on neuropsychiatric symptoms in Alzheimer's dementia: evidence from the CitAD study. Am J Psychiatry 173(5):473–480, 2016

Rabins PV, Mace NL, Lucas MJ: The impact of dementia on the family. JAMA 248(3):333–335, 1982

Reus VI, Fochtmann LJ, Eyler AE, et al: The American Psychiatric Association practice guideline on the use of antipsychotics to treat agitation or psychosis in patients with dementia. Am J Psychiatry 173(5):543–546, 2016

Sink KM, Holden KF, Yaffe K: Pharmacological treatment of neuropsychiatric symptoms of dementia: a review of the evidence. JAMA 293(5):596–608, 2005

Weiner MF, Lipton AM (eds): The American Psychiatric Publishing Textbook of Alzheimer Disease and Other Dementias. Washington, DC, American Psychiatric Publishing, 2009

Chapter 17

Personality Disorders

Personality disorders are an enduring pattern of inner experience and behavior that deviates markedly from the expectations of the individual's culture; is pervasive and inflexible; has onset in adolescence or early adulthood; is stable over time; and leads to distress or impairment. As a general rule, personality disorders represent long-term functioning and are not limited to episodes of illness. DSM-5 lists 10 personality disorders divided among three "clusters" (Table 17–1). Each cluster is characterized by phenomenologically similar disorders, or disorders whose criteria overlap.

- *Cluster A—paranoid, schizoid, and schizotypal personality disorders*—characterized by a pervasive pattern of abnormal cognition (e.g., suspiciousness), self-expression (e.g., odd speech), or relating to others (e.g., reclusiveness).
- *Cluster B—borderline, antisocial, histrionic, and narcissistic personality disorders*—characterized by a pervasive pattern of violating social norms or the rights of others (e.g., criminal behavior), impulsivity, excessive emotionality, grandiosity, or "acting out" (e.g., tantrums, self-abusive behavior, angry outbursts).
- *Cluster C—avoidant, dependent, and obsessive-compulsive personality disorders*—characterized by a pervasive pattern of abnormal fears involving social relationships, separation, and need for control.

General Issues

Epidemiology

Personality disorders are common and affect 9%–16% of the general population. The prevalence is even greater in hospital and clinic populations, among prisoners, and in those

TABLE 17–1. DSM-5 personality disorders

Cluster A (the "eccentric" disorders)

Paranoid

Schizoid

Schizotypal

Cluster B (the "dramatic" disorders)

Antisocial

Borderline

Histrionic

Narcissistic

Cluster C (the "anxious" disorders)

Avoidant

Dependent

Obsessive-compulsive

---

with substance use disorders. Antisocial personality disorder occurs more frequently in men, whereas borderline personality disorder, histrionic personality disorder, and dependent personality disorder are more frequent among women. Other personality disorders (e.g., schizoid, schizotypal, and obsessive-compulsive personality disorders) have a fairly equal gender distribution. Younger persons are at greater risk for a personality disorder than older individuals. Substance misuse and cigarette smoking are more frequent among those with a personality disorder than those without.

If a personality disorder is diagnosed in a person younger than 18 years, DSM-5 requires that the maladaptive personality features be present for at least 1 year. The exception is antisocial personality disorder, which has an age requirement of 18 years and requires that certain childhood behaviors be present along with the adult traits.

Personality disorders are associated with impaired social, interpersonal, and occupational adjustment; increased rates of health care utilization; and excessive rates of traumatic accidents. As a group, individuals with personality disorders are at risk for early death from suicide or accidents.

Personality disorders generally are thought of as stable and enduring. One recent follow-up study showed that many persons with a personality disorder (40%) no longer had a pattern of inner experience and behavior that met diagnostic criteria 2 years later. Persons with the poorest functioning initially tended to have the poorest functioning at follow-up. This study confirms that personality disorders become less symptomatic over time.

Comorbid mental disorders are common, including mood, anxiety, substance use, and eating disorders. Few persons have a "pure" case in which criteria for only a single personality disorder are met.

Importantly, the presence of a personality disorder often is associated with a poorer response to treatment, as has been shown for several mental disorders, including major depression, panic disorder, and obsessive-compulsive disorder.

Diagnosis

The patient's history forms the most important basis for diagnosing a personality disorder. For general screening purposes, a clinician might ask about problems with interpersonal relationships, the patient's sense of self, work, affect, impulse control, and reality testing. Suggested questions include the following:

- Do you often have days when your mood is constantly changing?
- How do you feel when you are not the center of attention?
- Do you frequently insist on having what you want right now?
- Are you concerned that certain friends or co-workers are not really loyal or trustworthy?
- Are you concerned about saying the wrong things in front of other people?
- How often do you avoid getting to know someone because you are worried he or she may not like you?

Collateral information is helpful especially when the patient denies—or seems unaware of—his or her maladaptive traits. Information from relatives or friends can help confirm the severity and pervasiveness of the individual's problems. Long-term observation might be necessary with some patients to confirm the diagnosis of personality disorder.

Treatment

Treatments for personality disorders can be divided into pharmacological and psychosocial. There are no FDA-approved medications for *any* personality disorder. Although in regard to medication, some personality disorders have been studied extensively (e.g., borderline personality disorder), others have been researched little or almost not at all (e.g., histrionic personality disorder). The same is true for psychotherapy. Borderline personality disorder has been actively studied, and several evidence-based psychotherapies now exist, but the other disorders have been virtually ignored. Treatment for each personality disorder will be discussed in the following section.

The DSM-5 Personality Disorders

Cluster A Disorders

Paranoid Personality Disorder

Paranoid personality disorder patients are chronically suspicious, distrust others, and fulfill their suspicious prophecies by leading others to be overly cautious and deceptive. Frank delusions are absent. Persons with paranoid personality disorder rarely seek treatment, likely because of their general mistrust of others. The disorder has an estimated prevalence of 1%–4% in the general population and often is first recognized when the patient seeks treatment for a mood or anxiety disorder.

Apart from diagnosing and treating the patient's comorbid disorders (e.g., major depressive disorder), the psychiatrist should be supportive and listen patiently to the patient's accusations and complaints while being open, honest, and respectful. When rapport has been established, alternative explanations for the patient's misperceptions can be suggested. Avoid group therapy because patients with paranoid personality disorder tend to misinterpret statements and situations that arise in the course of the therapy. Antipsychotics have been used off-label to reduce suspiciousness, but they have not been specifically studied for this condition.

Schizoid Personality Disorder

Schizoid personality disorder is a diagnosis used for patients with a profound defect in the ability to form personal relationships and to respond to others in a meaningful way. These patients have no close relationships—apart from with family members—and choose solitary activities. They rarely experience strong emotions, express little desire for sexual intimacy, are indifferent to praise or criticism, and display a constricted affect.

Schizoid personality disorder has a prevalence of 3%–5% in the general population. It is relatively uncommon in clinical settings because persons with this disorder rarely seek psychiatric care. There are no specific treatments for the disorder. People with this disorder generally come to clinical attention because of a comorbid disorder such as major depression. They tend to lack the insight and motivation necessary for individual psychotherapy and probably would find the intimacy of traditional group therapy threatening.

Schizotypal Personality Disorder

Schizotypal personality disorder is considered part of the schizophrenia spectrum, along with schizophreniform disorder, schizoaffective disorder, and schizophrenia. The disorder is characterized by a pattern of peculiar behavior, odd speech and thinking, and unusual perceptual experiences. Schizotypal patients frequently are socially isolated and have "magical" beliefs, mild paranoia, inappropriate or constricted affect, and social anxiety. Schizotypal personality disorder has a prevalence of approximately 4%–5%, and there is no gender difference. Comorbidity with mood, substance use, and anxiety disorders is common.

Treatment often centers on issues that led the person to seek treatment, such as feelings of alienation or isolation, paranoia, or suspiciousness. Exploratory and group psychotherapies might be overly threatening to these patients, but social skills training can be helpful. The goal is to help the individual develop an awareness of what behaviors others (e.g., coworkers) might consider odd or eccentric and develop a repertoire of social skills that will assist him or her in making interactions with others more productive and satisfying. Antipsychotics sometimes are used off-label to help reduce the intense anxiety, paranoia, and unusual perceptual experiences these individuals experience.

Cluster B Disorders

Antisocial Personality Disorder

Antisocial personality disorder is characterized by serial misbehavior that begins in childhood or early adolescence and continues into adulthood. Antisocial patients typically report a history of childhood behavior problems (e.g., fighting with peers, conflicts with adults) that fulfill criteria for conduct disorder. Fire setting and cruelty to animals and other children are particularly worrisome symptoms. As the antisocial youth reaches adulthood, other problems develop reflecting age-appropriate responsibilities, such as uneven job performance or domestic abuse. Unreliability, reckless behavior, and inappropriate aggression are frequent problems. Criminal behavior, pathological lying, and the use of aliases also are characteristic of the disorder. Marriages often are marked by instability or emotional and physical abuse of the spouse; separation and divorce are common. The DSM-5 criteria for antisocial personality disorder are shown in Box 17–1.

Box 17–1. DSM-5 Criteria for Antisocial Personality Disorder

A. A pervasive pattern of disregard for and violation of the rights of others, occurring since age 15 years, as indicated by three (or more) of the following:

1. Failure to conform to social norms with respect to lawful behaviors, as indicated by repeatedly performing acts that are grounds for arrest.
2. Deceitfulness, as indicated by repeated lying, use of aliases, or conning others for personal profit or pleasure.
3. Impulsivity or failure to plan ahead.
4. Irritability and aggressiveness, as indicated by repeated physical fights or assaults.
5. Reckless disregard for safety of self or others.
6. Consistent irresponsibility, as indicated by repeated failure to sustain consistent work behavior or honor financial obligations.
7. Lack of remorse, as indicated by being indifferent to or rationalizing having hurt, mistreated, or stolen from another.

B. The individual is at least age 18 years.
C. There is evidence of conduct disorder with onset before age 15 years.
D. The occurrence of antisocial behavior is not exclusively during the course of schizophrenia or bipolar disorder.

Antisocial personality disorder has a prevalence of 2%–4% in men and 0.5%–1% in women and is much more common in psychiatric hospitals and clinics, among the homeless and the incarcerated, and among substance-abusing persons. The disorder is worse early in its course, and antisocial symptoms tend to recede with age.

Comorbid substance use disorders, mood and anxiety disorders, attention-deficit/hyperactivity disorder, other personality disorders (e.g., borderline personality disorder), and gambling disorder are common. Antisocial persons frequently attempt suicide, and mortality studies show high rates of death from natural causes as well as accidents, suicides, and homicides.

The disorder has no standard treatment. Several medications have been used off-label to reduce aggression—the chief problem for many antisocial persons. They include lithium, valproate, and antipsychotics. Stimulants and benzodiazepines should be avoided because of their abuse potential; further, benzodiazepines can cause behavioral dyscontrol. Medication should target comorbid disorders, such as major depressive disorder. Cognitive-behavioral therapy (CBT) could help those with milder syndromes.

Borderline Personality Disorder

Borderline personality disorder is characterized by a pervasive pattern of unstable emotions, impulsivity, and disturbed relationships. Patients also might experience transient paranoid ideation or dissociative symptoms. The DSM-5 criteria for borderline personality disorder are shown in Box 17–2.

Box 17–2.   DSM-5 Criteria for Borderline Personality Disorder

---

A pervasive pattern of instability of interpersonal relationships, self-image, and affects, and marked impulsivity, beginning by early adulthood and present in a variety of contexts, as indicated by five (or more) of the following:

1. Frantic efforts to avoid real or imagined abandonment. (**Note:** Do not include suicidal or self-mutilating behavior covered in Criterion 5.)
2. A pattern of unstable and intense interpersonal relationships characterized by alternating between extremes of idealization and devaluation.
3. Identity disturbance: markedly and persistently unstable self-image or sense of self.

4. Impulsivity in at least two areas that are potentially self-damaging (e.g., spending, sex, substance abuse, reckless driving, binge eating). (**Note:** Do not include suicidal or self-mutilating behavior covered in Criterion 5.)
5. Recurrent suicidal behavior, gestures, or threats, or self-mutilating behavior.
6. Affective instability due to a marked reactivity of mood (e.g., intense episodic dysphoria, irritability, or anxiety usually lasting a few hours and only rarely more than a few days).
7. Chronic feelings of emptiness.
8. Inappropriate, intense anger or difficulty controlling anger (e.g., frequent displays of temper, constant anger, recurrent physical fights).
9. Transient, stress-related paranoid ideation or severe dissociative symptoms.

Borderline personality disorder has a prevalence in the general population of 1%–2%. More than three-quarters of borderline patients engage in deliberate self-harm (e.g., cutting, overdoses), and approximately 10% commit suicide. Better long-term outcome is associated with higher intelligence, self-discipline, and social support from friends and relatives. Hostility, antisocial behavior, suspiciousness, and vanity are associated with poor outcome. These patients frequently have comorbid major depressive disorder, dysthymia, anxiety disorders, and substance abuse or dependence.

Several group treatment programs have been developed that appear to lessen associated mood instability, impulsivity, and social disability. Dialectical behavior therapy (DBT) is the best-known program and involves intensive year-long treatment with both individual and group therapy. An alternative is the less intensive 20-week Systems Training for Emotional Predictability and Problem Solving (STEPPS) program that combines psychoeducation and skills training. There are other evidence-based programs, but all of them suffer from limited availability.

There are no FDA-approved medications for borderline personality disorder. Selective serotonin reuptake inhibitors (SSRIs) might be helpful in reducing depressive symptoms and suicidal behaviors. Antipsychotics can help treat perceptual distortions, anger dyscontrol, suicidal behavior, and mood instability. Because suicide attempts are frequent among these patients, physicians should be cautious about prescribing any medication that could be dangerous in overdose. Avoid benzodiazepines, except perhaps for short-term use (e.g., days to weeks), because they can cause behavioral disinhibition or could be abused.

Histrionic Personality Disorder

Histrionic personality disorder is characterized by a pattern of excessive emotionality and attention-seeking behavior. Typical symptoms include excessive concern with appearance and wanting to be the center of attention. Histrionic persons often are gregarious and superficially charming but can be manipulative, vain, and demanding.

The disorder has a prevalence of nearly 2% in the general population. Histrionic persons tend to seek out medical attention and make frequent use of available health services. Histrionic personality disorder has been linked with somatization disorder (now somatic symptom disorder) and antisocial personality disorder in family studies.

CBT has been used to help patients counter their distorted thinking, such as the inflated self-image that many histrionic patients have. With interpersonal psychotherapy, the patient can focus on conscious (or unconscious) motivations for seeking out disappointing partners and being unable to commit oneself to a stable, meaningful relationship. Group therapy may be useful in addressing provocative and attention-seeking behavior. Patients might not be aware of their annoying behaviors, and it could be helpful to have peers point them out.

Narcissistic Personality Disorder

Narcissistic personality disorder is characterized by grandiosity, lack of empathy, and hypersensitivity to evaluation by others. Narcissistic persons are egotistical, inflate their accomplishments, and often manipulate or exploit those around them to achieve their own aims. They have an exaggerated sense of entitlement and believe that they deserve special treatment. Narcissistic individuals often are irritating, haughty, or difficult; although they appear outwardly charming, relationships tend to be superficial and cold. They tend to have little insight into their own narcissism.

Narcissistic personality disorder has been considered uncommon, although one survey reported a prevalence of approximately 6%. Similar to other personality disorders, narcissistic personality disorder generally is viewed as stable over time, although research suggests that it may vary under the influence of significant life events, such as achievement and new relationships.

When these individuals seek help, it is likely for anger or depression they feel when deprived of something to which they feel entitled, such as a promotion. This is sometimes referred to as a "narcissistic injury." Treatment recommendations range from intensive psychodynamic psychotherapy to interpersonal or cognitive-behavioral psychotherapy.

Cluster C Disorders

Avoidant Personality Disorder

People with avoidant personality disorder are inhibited, introverted, and anxious. These individuals tend to have low self-esteem, are hypersensitive to rejection, are apprehensive and mistrustful, are socially awkward and timid, are uncomfortable and self-conscious, and fear being embarrassed or acting foolish in public. Many features of avoidant personality disorder are indistinguishable from those of social anxiety disorder, and the two disorders frequently overlap.

Several psychotherapeutic strategies have been developed for treating avoidant personality disorder. Group therapy could help the person overcome his or her social anxiety and develop interpersonal trust. Assertiveness and social skills training can be helpful, as can systematic desensitization to treat anxiety symptoms, shyness, and introversion. CBT can help correct dysfunctional attitudes (e.g., "I had better not open my mouth because I'll probably say something stupid"). Benzodiazepines used short-term can be useful while the patient is attempting to enter previously avoided social situations. SSRIs also could be helpful because they effectively treat social anxiety disorder.

Dependent Personality Disorder

Dependent personality disorder is characterized by a pattern of relying excessively on others for emotional support. The disorder has a prevalence of approximately 0.5% in the general population. It is common among persons with chronic medical or psychiatric disorders. Comorbid mood and anxiety disorders are frequent. Individuals with dependent personality have poor social and family ties, in part because their dependency on others promotes interpersonal conflicts that serve to drive people away.

CBT has been recommended as a way to encourage emotional growth, assertiveness, effective decision making, and independence. Some patients could benefit from more focused assertiveness training or social skills training.

Obsessive-Compulsive Personality Disorder

Obsessive-compulsive personality disorder is characterized by perfectionism and inflexibility associated with overconscientiousness and constricted emotions. It has an estimated prevalence of 1%–2% in the general population. Unlike other personality disorders, this disorder appears to be more common in those with higher levels of education and those in higher income brackets. Comorbidity with mood and anxiety disorders is frequent. Do not confuse obsessive-compulsive personality disorder with obsessive-compulsive disorder. Individuals with the latter are more willing to identify their symptoms as pathological, whereas individuals with obsessive-compulsive personality disorder tend to view many of their symptoms (e.g., collecting, perfectionism) as desirable.

CBT might help these individuals understand that the world is not made up of clearly defined black and white lines of rigidly held beliefs. SSRIs may be helpful in reducing the need for perfectionism and unnecessary ritualizing that sometimes develops.

Clinical Points for Personality Disorders

- Patients have enduring, long-term problems, and therapy might be long-term as well. Years of maladaptive behavior cannot be easily understood or reversed.

- Have a positive attitude! Personality disorders cause a great deal of pain and suffering to patients and those in their lives. Have empathy for them.

- Avoid becoming overinvolved, such as giving out your cell phone number or relating your personal problems to the patient. These behaviors are called "boundary" issues, which indicate that the lines separating the relationship between doctor and patient have become blurred.

- Establish ground rules for therapy (e.g., that the therapist is willing to see the person regularly, at a specified time).

- Spell out what the patient should do or whom the patient should call when he or she is in a crisis.

- Spell out the consequences of self-damaging acts (e.g., hospitalization, referral to another therapist).

- Seek support for yourself from peers or supervisors. Some patients with personality disorders can be a handful, and the therapist may need advice or consultation from time to time.

- Support groups can be enormously helpful to the patient, and referral to community-based organizations is essential.

Further Reading

Beck AT, Davis DD, Freeman A: Cognitive Therapy of Personality Disorders, 3rd Edition. New York, Guilford, 2015

Black DW: Bad Boys, Bad Men: Confronting Antisocial Personality Disorder (Sociopathy)—Revised and Updated. New York, Oxford University Press, 2013

Blum N, St John D, Pfohl B, et al: Systems Training for Emotional Predictability and Problem Solving (STEPPS) for outpatients with borderline personality disorder: a randomized controlled trial and 1-year follow-up. Am J Psychiatry 165(4):468–478, 2008

Cowdry RW, Gardner DL: Pharmacotherapy of borderline personality disorder: alprazolam, carbamazepine, trifluoperazine, and tranylcypromine. Arch Gen Psychiatry 45(2):111–119, 1988

Grant BF, Hasin DS, Stinson FS, et al: Prevalence, correlates, and disability of personality disorders in the United States: results from the national epidemiologic survey on alcohol and related conditions. J Clin Psychiatry 65(7):948–958, 2004

Gunderson JG, Stout RL, McGlashan TH, et al: Ten-year course of borderline personality disorder: psychopathology and function from the Collaborative Longitudinal Personality Disorders study. Arch Gen Psychiatry 68(8):827–837, 2011

Levy KN, Chauhan P, Clarkin JF, et al: Narcissistic pathology: empirical approaches. Psychiatr Ann 39:203–213, 2009

Lieb K, Zanarini MC, Schmahl C, et al: Borderline personality disorder. Lancet 364(9432):453–461, 2004

Linehan MM, Comtois KA, Murray AM, et al: Two-year randomized controlled trial and follow-up of dialectical behavior therapy vs therapy by experts for suicidal behaviors and borderline personality disorder. Arch Gen Psychiatry 63(7):757–766, 2006

Oldham JM, Skodol AE, Bender DS (eds): The American Psychiatric Publishing Textbook of Personality Disorders, 2nd Edition. Washington, DC, American Psychiatric Publishing, 2014

PART III

Special Topics

Chapter 18

Psychiatric Emergencies

Violent and Assaultive Behaviors

Although mental health professionals cannot make accurate long-term predictions about violence, certain elements of the clinical situation, including the patient's diagnosis and past behavior, can give an indication of the patient's potential for imminent violence, thereby allowing appropriate interventions. A patient's *history of violent behavior* probably is the *single best predictor* of future dangerousness.

Etiology and Pathophysiology

Alcohol use disorders are strongly associated with violence because alcohol can cause disinhibition, decrease perceptual and cognitive alertness, and impair judgment. Other substances of abuse, including cocaine and other stimulants, hallucinogens, phencyclidine (PCP), and sedative-hypnotics, also are associated with violence and aggression.

Childhood aggression is one of the strongest predictors of adult violence. Of special concern is the triad of fire setting, animal cruelty, and enuresis during childhood that is especially predictive of violence. Many adult perpetrators of abuse are themselves victims of childhood abuse. For some, violence has its roots in a chaotic home environment.

Patients with schizophrenia, mania, neurocognitive disorders (e.g., dementia, delirium), and substance use disorders are more likely to become violent than patients with other diagnoses or persons who are not mentally ill. Moreover, psychotic persons are more likely to commit violent acts than non-psychotic individuals. Brain-injured and intellectually disabled persons also have a higher risk of committing violent acts.

At a neurophysiological level, aggressive behavior has been associated with disturbed central nervous system serotonin function. Low levels of cerebrospinal fluid (CSF) 5-hydroxyindoleacetic acid (5-HIAA), a serotonin metabolite, are correlated with impulsive violence. Serotonin has been hypothesized to act as the central nervous system's natural policing mechanism, helping to keep impulsive and violent behavior in check.

Risk factors for violence are summarized in Table 18–1.

Assessing Risk for Violence

Risk assessment for violent behavior involves a review of pertinent clinical variables and requires a thorough psychiatric history and careful mental status examination. Even in routine assessments, ask patients:

- Have you ever thought of harming someone else?
- Have you ever seriously injured another person?
- What is the most violent thing you have ever done?

Predicting violence can be compared with weather forecasting. As in weather forecasting, assessment of violence risk becomes less accurate beyond the short term (i.e., 24–48 hours). Furthermore, similar to weather forecasts, risk assessments should be updated frequently.

When interviewing a violent or threatening patient, remain calm and speak softly. Questions should seem nonjudgmental ("You seem upset; perhaps you can tell me why you feel that way").

Have an easy escape route in case the patient becomes aggressive. Avoid towering over the patient. Preferably, both patient and clinician should be seated, allowing personal distance between the two. Avoid direct eye contact and try to project a sense of empathy and concern. Interview family members, friends, police, and others who have pertinent information about the patient.

A differential diagnosis should be based on the patient's history, physical examination, and mental status examination, and in some cases laboratory findings. Interventions generally are based on the diagnosis. For example, a violent patient with schizophrenia will need treatment with antipsychotic medication.

Managing the Violent Patient

Whether in the hospital or clinic, a violent patient presents an emergency. To ensure the safety of the patient and others, it is important to have enough staff who are well trained in *seclu-*

TABLE 18–1. Risk factors associated with violence

A history of violent acts

Inability to control anger

A history of impulsive behavior (e.g., recklessness)

Paranoid ideation or frank psychosis

Lack of insight in psychotic patients

Command hallucinations in psychotic patients

A stated desire to hurt or kill another person

Presence of schizophrenia or bipolar disorder

Presence of antisocial personality disorder or borderline personality disorder

Presence of a dementia, delirium, or alcohol or drug intoxication

---

sion and restraint techniques. Students and residents should remember that seclusion or restraint is considered an emergency safety measure that aims to prevent injury to the patient and others and is never used as punishment or for staff convenience.

Once a decision has been made to restrain or seclude the patient, a staff member (with appropriate back-up) should approach the patient after first clearing the area of other patients. The staff person should tell the patient that he or she is being secluded or restrained because of uncontrolled behavior and ask him or her to walk quietly to the seclusion area with or without underarm support. If the patient does not cooperate, each staff member should take a limb according to a plan agreed on beforehand. The patient is brought to the ground, with his or her head controlled to avoid biting. Restraints are applied. Specific techniques will vary by institution, but all aim to ensure safety for the patient and others.

Once secluded, the patient should be searched. Belts, pins, and other potentially dangerous items should be removed, and the patient should be dressed in a hospital gown. Tranquilizing medication—if needed—can be injected or taken orally if the patient is cooperative. With agitated patients, combine a high-potency antipsychotic with a benzodiazepine (e.g., haloperidol, 2–5 mg; lorazepam, 1–2 mg). The dose of both agents can be repeated every 30 minutes until the patient has calmed sufficiently. One-on-one observation of the patient by nursing staff is mandatory.

Clinical Points About Violent Patients

- Predicting violent behavior is difficult, even under the best circumstances, but violence often is associated with the following:

  - Alcohol or drug intoxication

  - Neurocognitive disorders, such as Alzheimer's disease, delirium, or traumatic brain injury

  - Psychotic disorders

  - "Acting out" personality disorders (e.g., antisocial personality disorder, borderline personality disorder)

- Approach the patient in a slow and tactful manner.

  - Do not appear threatening or provocative.

  - Use a soft voice, appear passive, and maintain interpersonal distance.

  - Allow for ready escape: never let the patient get between you and the door.

- Ask the patient what is wrong or why he or she feels angry.

- Most patients are willing to disclose their feelings.

- Remember that violent psychiatric patients need to be in the hospital, where their safety and the safety of others can be assured.

- Write down orders for violence precautions and seclusion or restraint orders, when applicable.

  - Carefully monitor the risk of violence and the presence of assaultive behaviors.

  - Document the assessment and plan and review them frequently.

- Treat the underlying condition vigorously.

- For outpatients, monitor the risk of violent behaviors at each contact; the patient (or family) should remove all firearms from the home.

  - Instruct family members to contact the local police (i.e., call 911) if violence erupts.

Suicide and Suicidal Behavior

Nearly 1% of the U.S. general population will die by suicide. It is the tenth most frequent cause of death for adults and the third leading cause of death for persons ages 15–24. Suicide rates are specific for age, gender, and race. Rates for men increase steadily with age and reach a peak after age 75 years. Rates for women are highest in the late 40s or early 50s. Nearly three times as many men take their lives as women, and whites are more likely than blacks to kill themselves. Approximately two-thirds of suicide completers are men. Most are more than 45 years old, white, and separated, widowed, or divorced.

Firearms are the most common method used to commit suicide in the United States, perhaps because guns are readily available and often are immediately lethal. Following in frequency are poisoning (i.e., a drug overdose), hanging, cutting, jumping, and other methods. Men are more likely than women to use violent methods, such as firearms or hanging. Women tend to use less violent means, such as poisoning by overdose.

Clinical Findings

Ninety percent or more of suicide completers have symptoms that meet criteria for a major psychiatric disorder; more than one-half are depressed. Substance use disorders affect nearly one-half of suicide completers; schizophrenia, anxiety disorders, and other mental illnesses are less common. Risk for suicide is much higher among psychiatric patients than controls. Approximately 10%–15% of persons hospitalized with mood disorders and around 10% of persons with schizophrenia will commit suicide.

Clinical factors associated with risk for suicide are summarized in Table 18–2.

Suicide Attempters

Suicide attempts are intentional acts of self-injury that do not result in death and are at least 5–20 times more frequent than suicides. Individuals who attempt suicide are three times more likely to be female and usually younger than age 35 years. They act impulsively, make provisions for rescue, and use ineffective means such as drug overdoses. Approximately 10% of suicide attempters eventually will kill themselves.

TABLE 18–2. Clinical factors associated with suicide risk

Being a psychiatric patient

Male gender, although the gender distinction is less important among psychiatric patients than in the general population

Age: risk increases as men age but peaks in the middle years for women

Being divorced, widowed, or single

Race: whites are at higher risk than nonwhites

Diagnosis: depression, alcohol use disorder, schizophrenia

History of suicide attempts

Expressing suicidal thoughts or developing plans for suicide

Recent interpersonal loss (especially among patients who abuse alcohol)

Feelings of hopelessness and low self-esteem

Timing: more frequent early in the post–hospital discharge period

Adolescents: a history of drug abuse and behavior problems

Assessing the Suicidal Patient

Be alert to the possibility of suicide in any psychiatric patient, especially those who are depressed or have a depressed affect. Focus assessment on vegetative signs and cognitive symptoms of depression, death wishes, suicidal ideation, and suicidal plans.

Remember common risk factors with a simple mnemonic: SAD PERSONS. The initials stand for **S**ex (male gender), **A**ge (older), **D**epression, **P**revious (suicide) attempt, **E**thanol abuse, **R**ational thinking loss, **S**ocial support lacking, **O**rganized plan, **N**o spouse, **S**ickness.

Suicidal patients generally are willing to discuss their thoughts and should be asked:

- Are you having any thoughts that life isn't worth living?
- Are you having any thoughts about harming yourself?
- Are you having any thoughts about taking your life?
- Have you developed a plan for committing suicide? If so, what is your plan?

Assess the patient's history of suicidal behavior by asking:

- Have you ever had thoughts of killing yourself?
- Have you ever attempted suicide? If so, would you tell me about the attempt?

Approach the topic of suicide in a slow and tactful manner, after developing rapport with the patient. Because suicidal thoughts can fluctuate, physicians should reassess suicide risk during each contact with the patient.

Managing the Suicidal Patient

Patients with well-developed plans and the means to carry them out require protection, usually on a locked psychiatric unit. If the suicidal patient refuses admission, it may be necessary to obtain a court order.

Nursing staff should remove sharp objects, belts, and other potentially lethal items from the patient. Some patients may need one-to-one observation with a nurse sitting next them at all times. Once the patient's safety has been ensured, treating the underlying illness can begin. Treatment will depend on the diagnosis. Among medications, only lithium and clozapine have been associated with lowered rates of suicide. Electroconvulsive therapy often is recommended for treating major depressive disorder in suicidal individuals because it has a quicker onset of action than medication.

Close follow-up is mandatory and should include frequent physician visits to assess mood and suicide risk as well as to provide psychotherapeutic support. Consider prescribing antidepressants with a high therapeutic index that are unlikely to be fatal in overdose, such as a selective serotonin reuptake inhibitor (SSRI). Family members can help monitor the patient's medication use. Importantly, instruct the family to remove all firearms from the home.

Clinical Points About Suicidal Patients

- Always ask depressed patients about suicidal thoughts and plans. You will not plant ideas that were not there merely by asking.

- Reassess and document suicidality at every visit with depressed patients.

- Some suicidal patients should be hospitalized, even if it is against their will. Patients who do not have suicidal plans probably can be managed at home provided that they have supportive families who are willing to watch them carefully.

- In the hospital, "suicide precautions" should be written in the doctors' orders; one-to-one nursing observation will be needed for some patients.

  - Carefully document signs and symptoms of depression and suicidality.

- Frequently monitor suicidality in outpatients. Antidepressants with a high therapeutic index, such as SSRIs or one of the newer antidepressants (e.g., bupropion, mirtazapine, duloxetine, venlafaxine), are preferred.

  - Family members should remove all firearms from the home.

- Even though risk factors are known, it is not possible to predict who will commit suicide.

  - Use good clinical judgment, provide close follow-up, and prescribe effective treatments.

Further Reading

Bostwick JM, Pabbati C, Geske JR, McKean AJ: Suicide attempt as a risk factor for completed suicide: even more lethal than we knew. Am J Psychiatry 173(11):1094–1100, 2016

Coryell W, Young EA: Clinical predictors of suicide in primary major depressive disorder. J Clin Psychiatry 66(4):412–417, 2005

DeVylder JE, Lukens EP, Link BG, Lieberman JA: Suicidal ideation and suicide attempts among adults with psychotic experiences: data from the Collaborative Psychiatric Epidemiology Surveys. JAMA Psychiatry 72(3):219–225, 2015

Dolan M, Doyle M: Violence risk prediction. Clinical and actuarial measures and the role of the Psychopathy Checklist. Br J Psychiatry 177:303–311, 2000

Ferguson SD, Coccaro EF: History of mild to moderate traumatic brain injury and aggression in physically healthy participants with and without personality disorder. J Pers Disord 23(3):230–239, 2009

Mann JJ, Ellis SP, Waternaux CM, et al: Classification trees distinguish suicide attempters in major psychiatric disorders: a model of clinical decision making. J Clin Psychiatry 69(1):23–31, 2008

McNiel DE, Chamberlain JR, Weaver CM, et al: Impact of clinical training on violence risk assessment. Am J Psychiatry 165(2):195–200, 2008

Patterson WM, Dohn HH, Bird J, Patterson GA: Evaluation of suicidal patients: the SAD PERSONS scale. Psychosomatics 24(4):343–345, 348–349, 1983

Pulay AJ, Dawson DA, Hasin DS, et al: Violent behavior and DSM-IV psychiatric disorders: results from the national epidemiologic survey on alcohol and related conditions. J Clin Psychiatry 69(1):12–22, 2008

Simon RI: Preventing Patient Suicide: Clinical Assessment and Management. Washington, DC, American Psychiatric Publishing, 2011

Chapter 19

Legal Issues

Legal issues pertaining to mental illness can be divided into two broad categories:

- *Civil law,* which has to do with relationships between citizens
- *Criminal law,* which focuses on the individual's relationship to the state in the maintenance of social order

Civil issues pertinent to the practice of psychiatry include confidentiality, informed consent, and involuntary treatment. Criminal issues that might involve input from mental health practitioners include competence to stand trial (whether the person understands the court process and can assist his or her lawyer in the present) and criminal responsibility (whether the person accused of a crime was legally insane at the time of the act). Table 19–1 shows the distinction between civil and criminal laws pertaining to psychiatry.

This chapter focuses primarily on civil issues encountered by a psychiatrist during the course of his or her day-to-day practice. *Forensic psychiatry,* a subspecialty within psychiatry, focuses on the interface between psychiatry and the law that includes conducting evaluations of mental capacity, injury, and disability for agencies and courts.

Civil Issues

Involuntary Treatment

Psychiatrists have a responsibility to ensure the safety of their patients. Therefore, when a patient who is thought to be a threat to self or others refuses hospitalization, the psychiatrist will seek a court order for involuntary hospitalization.

Because civil commitment involves depriving a person of some of his or her constitutional rights on the basis of a men-

TABLE 19–1. Civil and criminal legal issues involving psychiatrists

Civil	Criminal
Involuntary hospitalization	Competency to stand trial
Confidentiality	Criminal responsibility
Informed consent	
Malpractice	

tal illness, most states carefully regulate the process in the belief that the courts are more objective in this balancing act than mental health providers. Most commitment laws invoke the concepts of mental illness, dangerousness, and disability. For civil commitment, these laws require the presence of mental illness, although the precise definition of *mental illness* differs from place to place. The law may specify the conditions considered to be a mental illness and require that the mental illness be *treatable* to qualify for civil commitment.

The concept of *dangerousness* usually requires that persons present an imminent danger to themselves or others (i.e., within the next 24 hours if not hospitalized). Because psychiatrists are unable to accurately predict dangerousness except in the most obvious situations, this requirement can be difficult to apply. The third element, *disability*, is a measure of the patient's inability to properly care for him- or herself because of mental illness. Some states use the phrase *gravely disabled* or similar language to suggest that a person is unable to take care of his or her personal grooming, maintain adequate hydration, and feed himself or herself.

Most states permit patients to be hospitalized on an emergency basis to allow for a more detailed evaluation and short-term psychiatric intervention. This is after someone who knows the person files a petition and medical certification of the need for emergency commitment. This period may range from 1 to 20 days, depending on the jurisdiction.

Civil commitments occur by court order after a judicial finding of mental illness and potential harm to self or others if the individual is released; they provide for continued involuntary hospitalization. There are a variety of legal protections for mentally ill persons facing involuntary commitment, including a timely court hearing after appropriate notice, ability to be present at all commitment proceedings, representation by an attorney, presentation of evidence by both sides, and privilege against self-incrimination (the right to refrain from saying anything that may make one seem ill). The burden of proof is on the petitioner to establish the reason for commitment, and the patient is guaranteed the right to appeal. Although the statutes differ, all states allow involuntary administration of psychotropic medication to some extent.

Much litigation has concerned the right of civilly committed patients to refuse psychotropic medication in nonemergency situations. Antipsychotic medication has been the major focus of this litigation because of the risk of serious adverse effects such as *tardive dyskinesia*. Although the risks of treatment differ among these drugs (second-generation antipsychotics have a lower risk), some courts have emphasized the potential risk of treatment rather than its potential benefits. In some courts, treatment with antipsychotic medication has been elevated to the status of an "extraordinary" form of medical treatment requiring special scrutiny. In some states, a patient retains the right to refuse medication until the medical treatment team has petitioned the court to declare the patient incompetent to consent to or refuse medication. In other states, such as Iowa, psychiatrists are allowed to provide mental health treatment, including medication, to patients after a commitment order is issued.

In addition to involuntary inpatient treatment, most states (44 out of 50) have provisions for involuntary outpatient treatment. Such treatment might be employed when the patient is not quite ill enough to merit inpatient care but presents some risk of harm to self or others because of mental illness and will not voluntarily comply with outpatient treatment. Outpatient commitments can be helpful for improving treatment compliance and reducing the risk of rehospitalization.

Confidentiality

Maintaining confidentiality is one of the most important ethical and legal obligations that psychiatrists have to their patients. Before information is given to a third party, the patient must provide written consent except when disclosure is required by regulation or law.

The U.S. government, recognizing the importance of confidentiality of patient records, passed the Health Insurance Portability and Accountability Act (HIPAA). Under the privacy rule in HIPAA, health care providers could face fines and penalties if protected health information was released without informed consent except as required by law or as allowed by other parts of HIPAA.

In some situations, physicians are required by law to breach confidentiality to protect a vulnerable person from harm by a patient, such as in child or elder abuse. In these situations, the physician needs only to have a reason to believe that the abuse has occurred to trigger the reporting requirement.

The psychiatrist has a legal responsibility to protect the third party and can break confidentiality by notifying the threatened person and/or the police. This *duty to protect* is referred to as the *Tarasoff* rule, named after a 1976 California Supreme Court case. The court found that the therapist was responsible for harm when a patient revealed that he intended to hurt a third party. In that case, the therapist was aware of the potential threat but did not warn or protect the victim.

Once the psychiatrist believes that a patient could harm others, hospitalization can be sought to further evaluate the patient and to protect the intended victim. When there is an imminent threat to an identified victim, protecting the endangered person could involve phoning the individual to report the threat even after the clinician has hospitalized the patient.

Confidentiality can be legally breached for other reasons. In some states, mental health providers can disclose confidential information to family members or others responsible for the patient's ongoing treatment without consent when it is thought to be in the patient's best interest. Utilization review groups, physician peer reviewers, and third-party payers can have access to hospital charts.

Informed Consent

Obtain informed consent from all patients before any psychiatric treatment. Formal written consent is common in hospitals but is relatively unusual in small private offices. Inform patients of the indications and contraindications for the treatment, possible adverse effects, risk of no treatment, and alternative therapies (if applicable). Carefully document the results of the discussion. When the patient is not capable of giving consent, he or she should have a court-appointed guardian who can make health care decisions on his or her behalf. Many hospitals also require written informed consent for some treatments, such as psychotropic medications or electroconvulsive therapy (ECT).

Malpractice

Malpractice is negligence in the conduct of one's professional duties. Psychiatrists tend to be sued less frequently than other physicians. One reason is because psychiatrists, by virtue of the disorders treated and the types of treatments provided, are less likely to physically harm a patient.

The following are reasons why psychiatrists are sued:

- *Patient suicide.* Potential errors by a psychiatrist include failure to take an adequate history of suicidal behavior, provide adequate protection in the hospital, or communicate changes in the patient's condition to other doctors and nurses.
- *Failure to obtain informed consent.* Patients could claim that the information provided was inadequate, alternatives were omitted, or consent was never obtained.
- *Injuries from psychotropic medications.* Situations that have led to claims include failure to disclose relevant information to the patient about adverse effects (e.g., tardive dyskinesia), failure to obtain an adequate history, and prescribing a drug or drug combination when it is not indicated or when potentially harmful drug interactions might occur.
- *Patient abandonment. Abandonment* is defined as improperly terminating a doctor–patient relationship despite the continuing need for treatment. Abandonment can lead to legal actions for both negligence and breach of contract. To avoid litigation, the best course is to notify the patient of termination in writing and provide sufficient time for the patient to find another psychiatrist.
- *ECT.* Claims involving ECT are relatively rare but do occur and involve allegations of failure to obtained informed consent, inappropriate or improper treatment, or injury resulting from treatment, such as memory loss. Liability can be minimized by using ECT in accordance with accepted practice standards and monitoring and supervising patients carefully between treatments. Fully document the consent process.
- *Sexual activity with current or former patients.* A psychiatrist could be expelled from professional associations, have his or her license suspended or revoked, and even face criminal charges for such "boundary violations."

Criminal Issues

The two most common criminal issues that psychiatrists are asked to comment on are *competency to stand trial* and *criminal responsibility*. To receive a fair trial, a person must be able to understand the nature of the charges against him or her, the possible penalty, and the legal issues and procedures. He or she also must be able to work with the attorney in preparing a defense. The presence of a mental illness, even psychosis, generally does not render the defendant incompetent to stand trial.

Competence to stand trial is a legal—not a medical—determination. A judge makes this determination according to national standards established by the U.S. Supreme Court in *Dusky v. United States* (1960). When the court determines that the defendant is incompetent to stand trial, the individual typically is transferred to a psychiatric hospital for treatment focused on restoring him or her to a competent state. Once competency has been restored, the defendant is returned to court to stand trial. Importantly, competence to stand trial refers to the "here and now" assessment of the person's ability to understand the nature of the proceedings and to assist council, regardless of the presence of mental illness.

Criminal responsibility, by contrast, has to do with the individual's state of mind at the time of a crime (i.e., "there and then"). Under our current system, a crime is considered to occur only when both bad behavior (*actus rea*) and a blameworthy state of mind (*mens rea*) are present. A person might be so mentally ill that he or she lacks this blameworthy state of mind by virtue of the disorder. In such a case, a person is said to lack criminal responsibility and is adjudicated as not guilty by reason of insanity. In practice, a successful insanity defense is rare.

Not all states have an insanity defense, and those that do use different standards for determining criminal responsibility. According to the widely accepted *M'Naghten* standard—modifications of which are used in many states—the person seeking the insanity defense must show that he or she had a mental illness that was so symptomatic that it left him or her unable to know the nature and quality of the act or unable to know that the act was wrong at the time of the alleged offense.

Even severely symptomatic patients will only rarely meet the insanity standard. Depending on the jurisdiction, other defenses such as diminished capacity and "guilty but mentally ill" can be used. In diminished capacity, the person is said to be unable to form intent to commit the crime he or she was charged with, but may be found guilty of a lesser charge. In the case of guilty but mentally ill, the person is said to lack the capacity to conform his or her behavior to the requirements of the law at the time of the act despite knowing that the act was wrong. Defendants found "guilty but mentally ill" usually are sentenced to correctional facilities and receive a psychiatric evaluation and appropriate treatment if indicated.

Clinical Points About Legal Issues

- In seeking involuntary hospitalization for a patient, there must be evidence of a treatable mental illness, imminent harm to self or others, or grave disability.

  - Become familiar with local and state laws.

  - Know the local judge or magistrate who handles civil commitments.

  - Outpatient commitments are useful in seriously mentally ill patients who are chronically noncompliant with treatment.

- Understand applicable state laws on confidentiality and informed consent.

- Breaching confidentiality under the *Tarasoff* rule could involve contacting the threatened third party.

- Malpractice lawsuits are common in our litigious society; adequate insurance is essential.

  - The best defense against successful claims of malpractice is to maintain proper documentation.

- Most psychiatrists do not routinely conduct competency evaluations to determine whether a patient can stand trial. Psychiatrists should get to know their forensic psychiatrist peers.

Further Reading

Appelbaum PS: Clinical practice. Assessment of patients' competence to consent to treatment. N Engl J Med 357(18):1834–1840, 2007

Appelbaum PS, Gutheil TG: Clinical Handbook of Psychiatry and the Law, 4th Edition. Philadelphia, PA, Lippincott Williams & Wilkins, 2007

Buchanan A: Competency to stand trial and the seriousness of the charge. J Am Acad Psychiatry Law 34(4):458–465, 2006

Frank B, Gupta S, McGlynn DJ: Psychotropic medications and informed consent: a review. Ann Clin Psychiatry 20(2):87–95, 2008

Giorgi-Guarnieri D, Janofsky J, Keram E, et al; American Academy of Psychiatry and the Law: AAPL practice guideline for forensic psychiatric evaluation of defendants raising the insanity defense. J Am Acad Psychiatry Law 30 (2, suppl):S3–S40, 2002

Gold LH, Frierson RL (eds): The American Psychiatric Association Publishing Textbook of Forensic Psychiatry, 3rd Edition. Washington DC, American Psychiatric Association Publishing, 2018

Gutheil TG, Gabbard GO: Misuses and misunderstandings of boundary theory in clinical and regulatory settings. Am J Psychiatry 155(3):409–414, 1998

Mossman D, Noffsinger SG, Ash P, et al; American Academy of Psychiatry and the Law: AAPL Practice Guideline for the forensic psychiatric evaluation of competence to stand trial. J Am Acad Psychiatry Law 35 (4, suppl):S3–S72, 2007

Simon RI, Gold LH (eds): Textbook of Forensic Psychiatry. Washington, DC, American Psychiatric Publishing, 2004

Simon RI, Shuman DW: Clinical Manual of Psychiatry and Law. Washington, DC, American Psychiatric Publishing, 2007

Chapter 20

Psychotherapy

Because psychiatrists deal with disorders that involve thoughts, feelings, and relationships, it is essential that clinicians become skilled using therapies directed at the mind in addition to the brain, collectively referred to as *psychotherapy*. For some disorders, such as borderline personality disorder, psychotherapies are first-line treatments. For many other disorders, such as bipolar disorder, they are an important adjunct to medications by encouraging treatment adherence, educating patients about their disorder, and providing insight or support to deal with the psychological consequences of having a major mental disorder.

This chapter provides a brief overview of the major classes of psychotherapy. These include individual psychotherapy, including behavior therapy and cognitive-behavioral therapy (CBT); group therapy; couples therapy; family therapy; and social skills training (see Table 20–1).

Individual Psychotherapy

The term *individual psychotherapy* covers a range of psychotherapeutic techniques, wherein a single therapist works with a single patient. Although there are many types of psychotherapy, the description provided here is a simplified and selective overview. Although developers of psychotherapy emphasize their differences, in fact most share common elements (Table 20–2).

Supportive Psychotherapy

Supportive psychotherapy is the most common individual psychotherapy and is used to help patients get through difficult situations. Components of supportive psychotherapy can be incorporated into any other type of psychotherapy. With supportive psychotherapy, the therapist maintains an attitude of sympathy, interest, and concern. Patients describe and discuss problems they are confronting, which could range

TABLE 20–1. Types of psychotherapy

Individual therapy

  Supportive psychotherapy

  Behavior therapy

  Cognitive-behavioral therapy

  Acceptance and commitment therapy

  Psychoanalysis

  Psychodynamic psychotherapy

  Insight-oriented psychotherapy

  Relationship psychotherapy

  Interpersonal psychotherapy

Group therapy

Couples therapy

Family therapy

Social skills training

from marital discord to psychotic experiences such as perse-cutory delusions. The therapist counters with encouragement and even specific advice. Supportive psychotherapy is appropriate for the full range of mental disorders, from adjustment disorders to the psychoses and even dementia.

The therapist could suggest that patients develop new interests or hobbies, try new activities that may expand their range of social contacts, achieve emancipation from their parents by moving into independent living circumstances, or even develop more organized study habits to improve school performance. Psychotic patients could be taught to refrain from discussing their delusional ideas, except with the therapist. Patients who abuse alcohol may receive praise and encouragement for refraining from drinking as well as suggestions about ways to increase self-esteem by achieving mastery and control, such as through improving skills in a sport or developing a new creative hobby. Methods commonly used in supportive psychotherapy are shown in Table 20–3.

Behavior Therapy

Behavior therapy is particularly helpful for disorders associated with disturbed behavior patterns, such as substance use

TABLE 20–2. Common elements among psychotherapies

Based on an interpersonal relationship

Use of verbal communication between two (or more) people as a healing element

Therapist's specific expertise in using communication and relationships in a healing way

Based on a rationale or conceptual structure that is used to understand the patient's problems

Use of a specific procedure in the relationship that is linked to the rationale

Structured relationship (e.g., contact time, frequency, and duration are prespecified)

Expectation of improvement

TABLE 20–3. Methods commonly used in supportive psychotherapy

Conversational style

Praise, reassurance, and encouragement

Advice

Rationalization and reframing

Rehearsal or anticipatory guidance

Confrontation, clarification, and interpretation

---

disorders, eating disorders, anxiety disorders, phobias, and obsessive-compulsive disorder. Techniques focus on *what the patient does*. The motto for this approach is "Change the behavior and the feelings will follow."

Although a detailed discussion of behavior therapy is beyond the scope of this book, learners will find it helpful to know some elements of behavior therapy including relaxation training, exposure, flooding, behavioral activation, and behavior modification.

Relaxation Training

Relaxation training teaches patients to control their bodies and mental states. Patients learn how to achieve voluntary control over their feelings of tension and relaxation. Relaxation training can entail simply giving patients an instructional audio recording that they can listen to in order to practice the techniques on their own. During *progressive muscle relaxation,* the individual is instructed to systematically proceed through each major muscle group, learning to tense and then relax the muscles. Relaxation often is paired with *rebreathing* techniques that emphasize slow, deep breathing.

Exposure

Exposure requires that patients place themselves in situations that they usually avoid, in the interest of reducing the adaptive difficulties that result from their disorder. For example, patients with phobias learn that they should *expose themselves to what they are avoiding.* The therapist might ask a patient with agoraphobia to imagine what it is like to leave his or her house and visit a shopping mall where he or she typically develops panic attacks, thereby leading the patient to experience the attack. This is called *imaginal exposure* because it takes place in one's imagination. The patient gradually will become able to enter the feared situation—for example, entering a shopping mall—and use relaxation techniques while in the setting. This is called *in vivo exposure* because exposure involves a real situation. For persons with obsessive–compulsive disorder, exposure typically is paired with *response prevention,* often referred to as *ERP.* With this technique, the person is prevented from carrying out his or her usual behavioral response. For example, a person might be asked to touch a "contaminated" object such as a door knob, and then be asked not to wash his or her hands.

Flooding

Flooding involves teaching patients to extinguish anxiety produced by a feared stimulus by placing them in *continuous contact* with the stimulus and helping them learn that the stimulus does not in fact lead to any feared consequences. For example, a patient with a disabling fear of flying might need to take repeated flights until the fear is extinguished.

Behavioral Activation

Many mental disorders are characterized by inflexible narrowing of the patient's behavioral repertoire. For example, depressed patients frequently expect negative, painful outcomes in their daily lives and begin to constrict their lives to avoid such outcomes. *Behavioral activation*, also a component of cognitive therapy, seeks to reengage the patient in activities, big and small, and aims to reverse their withdrawal and isolation, thereby promoting rapid restoration of functioning.

Behavior Modification

Behavior modification techniques tend to use the concept of reinforcement as a way of shaping behavior—in particular, to reduce or eliminate undesirable behaviors and replace them with healthier behaviors or habits. Behavior modification techniques are especially appropriate for disorders characterized by poor impulse control, such as substance use disorders and eating disorders. Individual programs can be designed to suit the patient's unique needs by using stimuli that support and reinforce the new, healthier behaviors. A program for a patient with anorexia nervosa could include positive reinforcers (e.g., special rewards or privileges) to promote a desired behavior such as eating three well-balanced meals per day, as well as negative reinforcers (e.g., restricted activity); in each case, the reinforcers have the goal of weight restoration.

Different mixtures of behavior modification techniques are required for different disorders. For example, a program comprising a different schedule of reinforcers and targets might be appropriate for an obese patient. Behavior modification programs for patients with substance use disorders are more likely to stress teaching an individual to understand the cues that trigger his or her craving, such as the pent-up irritation of a long day at work. Rather than dropping by a neighborhood bar in response, the patient is encouraged to substitute other positive reinforcers, such as dropping by a health club.

Cognitive-Behavioral Therapy

The theory and practice of CBT, developed mainly by Aaron T. Beck, are based on the assumption that *cognitive structures* or *schemas* shape the way people react and adapt to a variety of situations they encounter in their lives. Each person has his or her own specific set of cognitive structures that determines how he or she will react to any stressor in any particular situation. A person develops a psychiatric syndrome, such as anxiety or depression, when these schemas become overactive and predispose him or her to developing a pathological or negative response.

The most widespread use of CBT is for treating depression. In this example, the depressed individual typically has schemas that lead to *negative interpretations*. Beck described the three major cognitive patterns observed in depression as the cognitive triad:

- A negative view of oneself
- A negative interpretation of experience
- A negative view of the future

CBT has been adapted to treat anxiety disorders, eating disorders, obsessive-compulsive disorder, personality disorders, and many other conditions including insomnia. CBT focuses on teaching patients new ways to change these maladaptive schemas. CBT tends to be relatively short-term and highly structured. The goal is to help patients restructure their negative cognitions so that they can perceive reality in a less distorted way and learn to react accordingly.

CBT combines behavioral techniques with cognitive restructuring. The behavioral techniques include homework assignments and a graded program of activities designed to teach patients that their negative schemas are incorrect and that they are able to achieve small successes and interpret them as such. Cognitive techniques are designed to help the patient identify and correct the dysfunctional schemas that shape the patient's perception of reality. They involve identifying the cognitive distortions the patient is prone to make and *automatic thoughts* that intrude into the patient's consciousness and produce negative attitudes. Six typical cognitive distortions are listed in Table 20–4.

In addition to these erroneous interpretations, patients often are troubled with a variety of automatic thoughts that spontaneously intrude into their flow of consciousness. The specific automatic thoughts vary among individuals but involve negative themes of self-denigration and failure (e.g., "You're so stupid," "You never do anything right," "People wouldn't want to talk to you"). These thoughts pop up spontaneously and produce an accompanying dysphoria. Patients are encouraged to identify these automatic thoughts and learn ways to counteract them. Such techniques include replacing these automatic thoughts with positive counter-

TABLE 20–4. Cognitive distortions treated with cognitive-behavioral therapy

Distortion	Definition
Arbitrary inference	Drawing an erroneous conclusion from an experience
Selective abstraction	Taking a detail out of context and using it to denigrate the entire experience
Overgeneralization	Making general conclusions about overall experiences and relationships based on a single experience
Magnification and minimization	Altering the significance of specific events in a way that is structured by negative interpretations
Personalization	Interpreting events as reflecting on the patient when they have no relation to him or her
Dichotomous thinking	Seeing things in an all-or-none manner

thoughts, testing the hypotheses embedded in the thoughts through behavioral techniques, and identifying and testing the assumptions behind the thoughts.

The goal of the cognitive component of CBT is to identify and restructure the negative schemas that shape the patient's perceptions. The cognitive goal is achieved similarly to the behavioral goals: the patient is encouraged to do homework, complete assignments that identify the occurrence of dysfunctional cognitions, and steadily test and correct these cognitions. The therapist also reviews these aspects of the patient's diary and helps formulate an organized program for restructuring the dysfunctional cognitive sets, providing ample empathy and positive reinforcement.

Acceptance and Commitment Therapy

Acceptance and commitment therapy (ACT) is a newer therapy that has roots in CBT. ACT can be used in patients with a variety of mental disorders and physical conditions, such as major depressive disorder, anxiety disorders, and even migraine. The goal of ACT is to help individuals adapt to the pain, grief, and inevitable disappointments that are part of life by developing greater psychological flexibility. ACT promotes *acceptance* of what cannot be changed, while encouraging the person to cultivate the habit of *committing* to doing things in line with their identified hopes, values, and goals even in the face of their desire to avoid painful and troubling thoughts and emotions.

Psychoanalysis and Psychodynamic Psychotherapy

Classical psychoanalysis was developed by Sigmund Freud during the early twentieth century and arose from his experience attempting to treat patients with hysterical conversion symptoms, such as pain and paralysis. Now used only in specific situations and settings, Freud's work has contributed to a greater understanding of the mental mechanisms involved in defense, coping, and adaptation.

Psychodynamic psychotherapy uses many of these concepts, but in ways that make them more suitable for treating larger numbers of patients. Psychodynamic psychotherapy is used for patients with a variety of problems, including personality disorders, anxiety disorders, and mild depression. Psychodynamic psychotherapy typically is conducted face to face. The therapist aims to help the patient in a neutral but empathic way. The patient is encouraged to review early relationships with parents and significant others but also can focus on the present. As in classical psychoanalysis, the patient is expected to do most of the talking, while the psychodynamic psychotherapist occasionally interjects clarifications to help the patient understand the underlying dynamics that shape his or her behavior. Psychodynamic psychotherapy typically involves one or two sessions a week and could involve 2–5 years of treatment.

Insight-Oriented and Relationship Psychotherapy

Insight-oriented psychotherapy draws on many basic psychodynamic concepts but focuses even more on interpersonal relationships and here-and-now situations than purely psychodynamic psychotherapy does. Patients are typically seen once a week for 50 minutes. During the sessions patients are encouraged to review and discuss relationships, attitudes toward themselves, and early life experiences. The therapist maintains an involved and supportive attitude and occasionally assists patients with interpretations that will help them achieve insights.

In *relationship psychotherapy*, the therapist assumes a more active role. The stress is on achieving a corrective emotional experience, with the therapist serving as a loving and trustworthy surrogate parent who assists the patient who is confronting unrecognized needs and unresolved drives. The patient typically is seen once a week, and the therapy can last from 6 months to several years, depending on the patient's problems and maturity level. As in insight-oriented psychotherapy, the content of the sessions focuses primarily on current situations and relationships, with some looking backward to early life experiences. Although the patient can achieve insight, the most important component of this type of psychotherapy is the empathic and caring attitude of the therapist.

Interpersonal Psychotherapy

Interpersonal psychotherapy (IPT) is a specific type of psychotherapy developed for treating depression, although it potentially is useful for other conditions, such as bulimia nervosa and borderline personality disorder. IPT stresses working on improving interpersonal relationships. Emphasis is placed on the present rather than on the past. The therapist helps the patient identify specific problem areas that may be interfering with self-esteem and interpersonal interactions, usually involving four general domains: grief, interpersonal disputes, role transitions, and interpersonal deficits. After the exploration and identification process, the therapist works systematically with the patient to facilitate learning new adaptive behaviors and communication styles. IPT usually is conducted in weekly sessions, and the course of therapy lasts 3–4 months.

Group Therapy

Group therapy is a highly efficient way for clinicians to follow up with and monitor relatively large numbers of patients. There are many different kinds of group therapy, which vary depending on the individuals who compose the group, the problems or disorders that they are confronting, the setting in which the group meets, the type of role that the group leader takes, and the established therapeutic goals. Therapeutic mechanisms in group therapy are described in Table 20–5.

Group therapy programs have been established in many inpatient psychiatric hospitals. In very large inpatient hospitals, several groups could run concurrently and be composed of patients with similar types of problems. For example, one group might consist of patients with severe mood and psychotic disorders, and another group might have individuals with eating disorders. Such groups provide patients with a forum to share their problems; diminish their sense of isolation and loneliness; enable them to learn new techniques to cope with their problems, either through other patients or the group leader; and provide support, inspiration, and hope. These groups could transition to an outpatient setting where patients continue to consolidate and support the learning and skills that were developed in the inpatient setting.

Some groups are oriented largely toward providing support, which might or might not have a professional leader. Examples of such support groups include 12-step meetings such as Alcoholics Anonymous, groups composed of military veterans, or groups composed of individuals who have experienced a serious medical illness or difficult surgery (e.g., women who have had mastectomies). Such groups provide a forum for sharing information, giving encouragement and support, and instilling hope.

Group psychotherapy also could be done as an alternative—or a supplement—to individual psychotherapy. Groups typically are led by experienced therapists and conducted with a co-therapist. These groups aim to achieve goals similar to those of insight-oriented and interpersonal psychotherapy or cognitive therapy within the context of a group setting.

Several group therapy programs have been developed to treat patients with borderline personality disorder (BPD). The best-known program is *dialectical behavior therapy*, which combines group and individual therapy. The intensive 1-year program includes a mix of psychotherapeutic techniques including CBT and mindfulness meditation derived from Buddhist practice.

Couples Therapy

Couples therapy involves working with two people who see themselves as partners in a committed relationship to help

TABLE 20–5. Therapeutic mechanisms in group therapy

Instilling hope

Developing socializing skills

Using imitative behavior

Experiencing catharsis

Imparting information

Behaving altruistically by attempting to help other members of the group

Experiencing a corrective recapitulation of the primary family group, developing a sense of group cohesiveness

Diminishing feelings of isolation (universality)

Learning through feedback how one's behavior affects others (interpersonal learning).

them stabilize and improve their relationship. Depending on the partners' commitment, couples therapy has many variations. Ideally, both partners are willing and cooperative participants who seek change. Sometimes, however, couples therapy is sought because of a crisis: one of the partners might have lost interest in the relationship (and may or may not want to get out), whereas the other is hanging on tight and trying to save the relationship. In the latter instance, one possible outcome might be the decision to end the relationship, and therapy might become divorce mediation and counseling.

A therapist conducting couples therapy must take care to maintain an atmosphere of fairness, neutrality, and impartiality. Either partner could be particularly sensitive to the possibility that the therapist may take sides and treat him or her unfairly. The therapist's gender may seem significant to either partner, even though the therapist will feel quite comfortable with his or her ability to be impartial. Couples therapy typically begins with identifying the specific problem. Each partner is asked to identify areas in which he or she would like to see change in the other. The therapist then attempts to guide the couple in implementing changes in a gradual, graded way, attacking one problem at a time. Often couples benefit from discussing their hopes for and expectations of each other in the context of personal values, prior family experiences (i.e., gender role expectations, based on the behavior of their parents), and needs for intimacy and independence that occur within the context of a relationship.

Family Therapy

Family therapy tends to focus on the larger family unit—at a minimum, one parent and the child (in single-parent families), but more typically both parents and the child (or a parent and stepparent, two separated parents, other parental pairings depending on the family environment in which the child lives), or one or more parents and the child plus siblings. Typically, the child is brought in initially for treatment of a specific problem, such as school difficulties, oppositional behavior, delinquency, or aggression. Often, it rapidly becomes clear that these problems exist in the overall context of the family setting.

In family therapy, the therapist is not dealing with two potential equals but rather with a hierarchy in which parents are expected to assume some authority and responsibility for the behavior of their child. The degree of hierarchy in the family will vary depending on the age of the child. For adolescents and teenagers, one important problem is the stress that the "child's" growing independence is adding to this hierarchical structure.

Family therapy also could be used to help families in which at least one member has a serious mental illness, such as schizophrenia or major depressive disorder. It is important to work within the medical model and emphasize that the patient has an illness for which neither the patient nor the family can be considered responsible. This approach minimizes guilt, scapegoating, and castigation. Families that are hostile toward or critical of the patient (high expressed emotion) should be counseled on ways to reduce their intense emotions, which, if unchecked, can lead to relapse.

Social Skills Training

Social skills training is a specific type of psychotherapy that focuses on fostering the patient's abilities to relate with others and cope with the demands of daily life. It is used primarily for patients with severe mental illnesses, such as schizophrenia, that often results in marked impairment in social skills.

Social skills training can be initiated on an inpatient basis, but the bulk of the effort typically is done with outpatients because the long-term goal is to assist patients in learning to live in the real world. Social skills training can be done individually, but more typically is accompanied by some group work, and could occur in the context of day treatment or sheltered workshops.

The techniques of social skills training primarily are behavioral. Specific problems are identified and addressed in a sequentially integrated manner. Severely disabled patients might need help initially with grooming and hygiene. They could need encouragement to learn to shave or bathe daily, to keep their clothes laundered, and to eat regular meals. They also might need help learning how to approach other people and talk with them appropriately. At higher levels of functioning, they may need assistance learning how to apply for a job, complete job interviews, and relate to employers and coworkers.

Clinical Points for Psychotherapy

- Psychotherapy is a key component of comprehensive psychiatric care.

  - Psychotherapy is a first-line treatment for many disorders (e.g., borderline personality disorder).

  - Psychotherapy is an important treatment adjunct for many patients taking psychotropic medication.

  - Combined treatment (psychotherapy plus psychotropic medication) tends to produce the best outcomes.

- There are many different types of psychotherapy, but most share similar elements including development of a personal relationship with the therapist, using communication and relationships in a healing way, and conveying a sense of hope and expectation for improvement.

- Supportive therapy commonly is used to help patients get through difficult times by providing sympathy, encouragement, and even specific advice. This approach is within reach of all physicians, not just psychiatrists.

- With behavior therapy, the motto is, "Change the behavior, and the feelings will follow."

- CBT aims to change or restructure maladaptive cognitive schemas. Through homework and graded exercises, the patient learns to counter negative thoughts and behaviors that tend to promote and maintain psychiatric disorders, such as major depression.

- Psychodynamic psychotherapies focus on the patient's relationships, attitudes toward himself or herself, and early life experiences. The goal is to help the patient achieve insight into the development and persistence of his or her symptoms and behaviors in order to bring about needed change.

- Group therapy is an efficient way to deliver care to many patients at once. It provides a surrogate peer group in which patients can learn new ways to interact with others in a controlled environment.

  - Several programs have been developed specifically to treat borderline personality disorder and, although they are helpful, lack of availability limits their usefulness.

- Couples and family therapies focus on either a dyad (the couple) or the larger family unit to address specific problems. In either situation, it is essential for the therapist to maintain an atmosphere of fairness, neutrality, and impartiality.

Further Reading

Beck AT, Alford BA: Depression: Causes and Treatment, 2nd Edition. Philadelphia, University of Pennsylvania Press, 2008

Gabbard GO: Psychodynamic Psychiatry in Clinical Practice, 4th Edition. Washington, DC, American Psychiatric Press, 2005

Gabbard GO (ed): Textbook of Psychotherapeutic Treatments. Washington, DC, American Psychiatric Publishing, 2009

Hayes S, Strosahl K, Wilson K: Acceptance and Commitment Therapy: An Experimental Approach to Behavior Change. New York, Guilford, 1999

Hopko DR, Lejuez CW, Ruggiero KJ, Eifert GH: Contemporary behavioral activation treatments for depression: procedures, principles, and progress. Clin Psychol Rev 23(5):699–717, 2003

Keitner GI, Heru AM, Glick ID: Clinical Manual of Couples and Family Therapy. Washington, DC, American Psychiatric Publishing, 2010

Linehan MM: Cognitive-Behavioral Treatment for Borderline Personality Disorder. New York, Guilford, 1993

Sudak D: Cognitive Behavioral Therapy for Clinicians. Baltimore, MD, Lippincott Williams & Wilkins, 2006

Winston A, Rosenthal RN, Pinsker H: Learning Supportive Psychotherapy: An Illustrated Guide. Washington, DC, American Psychiatric Publishing, 2012

Yalom ID, Leszcz M: The Theory and Practice of Group Psychotherapy, 5th Edition. New York, Basic Books, 2005

Chapter 21

Somatic Treatments

The modern era of psychiatric treatment began with the introduction of electroconvulsive therapy (ECT) in the late 1930s, chlorpromazine and tricyclic antidepressants (TCAs) in the 1950s, benzodiazepines and stimulants in the 1960s, and lithium in 1970. More recently, these treatments were joined by the selective serotonin reuptake inhibitor (SSRI) antidepressants and the second-generation antipsychotics (SGAs). Medication has revolutionized the practice of psychiatry and has been instrumental in helping to alleviate suffering and improve the lives of millions.

Antipsychotics

Antipsychotics can be roughly broken down into two groups: the older, first-generation antipsychotics (FGAs) and the newer, second-generation antipsychotics (SGAs), or atypical antipsychotics. Antipsychotics are used to treat schizophrenia and bipolar disorder, but they also are prescribed off label to control aggressive behavior in patients with intellectually disability, borderline personality disorder, delirium, or other neurocognitive disorders. The most commonly used antipsychotics, their adverse effects, and their dosages are listed in Table 21–1.

Mechanism of Action

The potency of FGAs correlates closely with their affinity for the dopamine type 2 (D_2) receptor, blocking the effect of endogenous dopamine at this site. SGAs differ in that they are weaker D_2 receptor antagonists than FGAs but are potent serotonin type 2A (5-HT_{2A}) receptor antagonists and have significant anticholinergic and antihistaminic activity as well. Central 5-HT_{2A} receptor antagonism is believed to broaden the thera-

TABLE 21–1. Common antipsychotic agents

Category	Drug (trade name)	Sedation	Orthostatic hypotension	Anticholinergic effects	Extrapyramidal effects	Equivalent dosage, mg	Dosage range, mg/day
First-generation (typical) agents							
Phenothiazines							
Aliphatics	Chlorpromazine (Thorazine[a])	H	H	M	M	100	50–1,200
Piperazines	Fluphenazine (Prolixin[a])	L	L	L	VH	2	2–20
	Fluphenazine decanoate	L	L	L	VH	—[b]	12.5–50 mg q 2 wk
	Perphenazine (Trilafon[a])	L	L	L	H	10	12–64
	Trifluoperazine (Stelazine[a])	L	L	L	H	5	5–40
Thioxanthenes	Thiothixene (Navane[a])	L	L	L	H	5	5–60
Butyrophenones	Haloperidol (Haldol)	L	L	L	VH	2	2–60

TABLE 21–1. Common antipsychotic agents (*continued*)

Category	Drug (trade name)	Sedation	Orthostatic hypotension	Anticholinergic effects	Extrapyramidal effects	Equivalent dosage, mg	Dosage range, mg/day
Second-generation (atypical) agents							
	Aripiprazole (Abilify)	L	VL	L	VL	7.5	10–15
	Asenapine (Saphris)	L	M	L	VL	5	10–20
	Cariprazine (Vraylar)	L	L	L	L	?	1.5–6
	Clozapine (Clozaril)	H	H	H	VL	100	200–600
	Lurasidone (Latuda)	L	L	L	VL	40	40–160
	Olanzapine (Zyprexa)	L	L	M	L	5	15–30
	Quetiapine (Seroquel)	M	L	L	VL	75	300–500
	Paliperidone (Invega)	L	M	L	L	4	3–12
	Risperidone (Risperdal)	L	M	L	L	2	2–6
	Ziprasidone (Geodon)	M	L	VL	L	60	40–160

Note. H=high; L=low; M=moderate; VH=very high; VL=very low.
[a]Brand no longer available in the United States.
[b]Long-acting ester; dosage is not directly comparable with that of standard compounds.

peutic effect of the drug while reducing the incidence of extra-pyramidal side effects (EPS) associated with D_2 antagonists.

Pharmacokinetics

Oral absorption of antipsychotics is variable, and peak plasma levels generally are reached in 1–4 hours. Injectable antipsychotics have much greater bioavailability than oral medication and work much more quickly. Metabolism occurs mostly in the liver, largely by oxidation, so that these highly lipid-soluble agents are converted to water-soluble metabolites and excreted in the urine and feces. Excretion of antipsychotics tends to be slow because of drug accumulation in fatty tissue. Most of the FGAs are highly protein bound (85%–90%). Nearly all antipsychotics have a half-life of 24 hours or longer and have active metabolites with longer half-lives. Depot formulations have even longer half-lives and may take 3–6 months to reach steady state.

Most FGAs are metabolized by the cytochrome P450 (CYP) enzyme subfamilies, including 2D6, 1A2, and 3A4. Because of genetic variation, 5%–10% of whites poorly metabolize medications through the CYP2D6 pathway, as do a significant portion of blacks. This can result in higher antipsychotic blood levels than anticipated in some patients.

Blood plasma levels of haloperidol and clozapine are helpful in determining treatment effectiveness. With haloperidol, optimal response is associated with serum concentrations of 5–15 ng/mL. With clozapine, levels >350 ng/mL appear to be effective. Other situations in which blood plasma levels are useful include the following:

- When patients' symptoms have not responded to standard dosages
- When antipsychotic medications are combined with drugs that can affect their pharmacokinetics (e.g., carbamazepine)
- When patient compliance needs to be assessed

Acute Treatment of Psychosis

A high-potency FGA (e.g., haloperidol, 5–10 mg/day) or an SGA (e.g., risperidone, 4–6 mg/day) is recommended as an initial choice. Antipsychotic effects generally start within days but are cumulative over the ensuing weeks. An adequate trial should last 4–6 weeks and extend for another 4–6 weeks if the patient shows a partial response. If no response occurs after 4–6 weeks, try a different drug. Clozapine is a second-line choice because it can cause agranulocytosis and requires monitoring of white blood cell count.

Highly agitated patients should receive frequent, equally spaced doses of an antipsychotic drug to control symptoms. High-potency antipsychotics (e.g., haloperidol, olanzapine) can be given every 30–120 minutes orally or intramuscularly until agitation has subsided. A combination of an antipsychotic and a benzodiazepine (e.g., haloperidol 5 mg, lorazepam 2 mg) might work better, with the doses repeated every 30 minutes until adequate tranquilization is achieved.

Maintenance Treatment

Long-term maintenance treatment aims to achieve sustained control of psychotic symptoms and reduce the risk of relapse. The following guidelines were developed at an international conference:

1. Prevention of relapse is more important than risk of adverse effects because most adverse effects are reversible, however the consequences of relapse may be irreversible.
2. At least 1–2 years of treatment are recommended after the initial episode because of the high risk of relapse and the possibility of social deterioration with further relapses.
3. At least 5 years of treatment are indicated for multi-episode patients.

Chronic, or ongoing, treatment is recommended for patients who pose a danger to themselves or others.

Adverse Effects

The severity of adverse effects from antipsychotics differs from drug to drug and corresponds with the drug's ability to affect specific neurotransmitters (see Table 21–1).

Extrapyramidal Side Effects

- *Tardive dyskinesia* (TD) consists of abnormal involuntary movements of the mouth and tongue, but other parts of the body can be affected. Movements generally are mild, but some patients have disabling symptoms. The preferred strategy is to stop the offending agent, but many patients will choose to continue taking the drug because their lives may be intolerable without medication. One option is to switch the patient to an SGA to mask the symptoms. Vitamin E could alleviate TD movements to a degree. The FDA recently approved valbenazine (Ingrezza) and deutetrabenazine (Austedo) to treat TD.

- *Akathisia*, the most common form of EPS, could appear soon after initiation of antipsychotic treatment. This condition causes subjective feelings of anxiety/tension and objective fidgetiness and agitation. The clinician could first reduce the drug dosage if possible, and then add a beta-blocker or amantadine. Benzodiazepines also help relieve akathisia symptoms.

- *Pseudoparkinsonism* usually takes 3 weeks or more to develop. Patients develop symptoms typical of Parkinson's disease, including tremor, rigidity, and hypokinesia. The clinician could first reduce the antipsychotic dosage if possible, and then consider adding an antiparkinsonian agent.

- *Acute dystonic reaction*, which usually occurs during the first 4 days of treatment, involves sustained contraction of the muscles of the neck, mouth, tongue, or occasionally other muscle groups that is distressing and often painful. Acute dystonias typically respond within 20–30 minutes to intramuscular benztropine or diphenhydramine.

Anticholinergic Adverse Effects

Dry mouth, urinary retention, blurry vision, constipation, and exacerbation of narrow-angle glaucoma are commonly caused by low-potency FGAs (e.g., chlorpromazine). These symptoms are best treated by reducing the dosage or switching to a more potent agent (e.g., haloperidol) or an SGA.

Orthostatic Hypotension

Orthostatic hypotension is mediated by α-adrenergic blockade. This adverse effect often is caused by low-potency drugs (e.g., chlorpromazine).

QTC Prolongation

Chlorpromazine, thioridazine, pimozide, and the SGAs aripiprazole and iloperidone have been associated with this adverse effect that can lead to abnormal cardiac conduction or sudden death.

Agranulocytosis

Agranulocytosis occurs in 0.8% of patients taking clozapine during the first year of treatment and peaks in incidence at 3 months of treatment.

Hyperprolactinemia/Gynecomastia

Galactorrhea (milk production) and gynecomastia in men are most likely to occur with risperidone and high-potency FGAs. SGAs—specifically quetiapine and aripiprazole—are less likely to cause hyperprolactinemia (prolactin is responsible for the condition). If it is not possible to reduce the dosage or change antipsychotics, bromocriptine could be helpful.

Metabolic Abnormalities

SGAs are associated with abnormalities in glucose regulation, lipids, and weight gain. Clozapine and olanzapine are most likely to cause weight gain, followed by risperidone and quetiapine. Aripiprazole, lurasidone, and ziprasidone are relatively weight neutral.

Neuroleptic Malignant Syndrome

Neuroleptic malignant syndrome (NMS) is a rare, idiosyncratic reaction that causes rigidity, high fever, delirium, and marked autonomic instability. Serum levels of creatine phosphokinase and liver enzymes generally are elevated. The antipsychotic should be discontinued and supportive care provided. Dantrolene and bromocriptine have been used to treat NMS, as has ECT.

Pregnancy

All antipsychotics except clozapine are listed as Category C by the FDA, meaning that risk to the fetus cannot be ruled out. Clozapine is listed as Category B, meaning that there is no evidence of fetal risk in humans.

Rational Use of Antipsychotics
1. Use a high-potency typical antipsychotic or an SGA as first-line treatment.
• SGAs are effective and well tolerated and are less likely to induce EPS.

2. Second-line drug choices include the other typical antipsychotics.

3. A drug trial should last 4–6 weeks.

    • The trial should be extended when there is a partial response that has not plateaued and shortened when no response occurs or side effects are intolerable or unmanageable.

    • Aripiprazole, ziprasidone, or lurasidone might be better choices in patients at risk for weight gain.

    • Quetiapine or aripiprazole could be favored when low EPS and low prolactin levels are desired.

4. Start all antipsychotics at a low dosage and gradually increase to fall within a therapeutic range.

    • Evidence suggests that blood levels can help guide dosage adjustments for haloperidol and clozapine.

5. There is little reason to prescribe more than one antipsychotic agent. Using two or more such drugs increases adverse effects and adds little clinical benefit.

6. Because of the risk of agranulocytosis and need for monitoring of the white blood cell count with clozapine, reserve clozapine for patients with treatment-refractory illness.

    • The FDA requires that patients must have an absolute neutrophil count of ≥1,500 μL to start clozapine and ≥1,000 μL to continue. Monitor CBCs and absolute neutrophil counts weekly for 6 months, every 14 days for another 6 months, and monthly thereafter.

7. Many patients can benefit from chronic SGA administration.

    • Consider measuring baseline body mass index (BMI), waist circumference, blood pressure, and fasting glucose and lipid panels. Then, follow BMI monthly for 3 months and then quarterly. Monitor blood pressure, fasting glucose, and lipid panels at 3 months and then yearly.

Antidepressants

Antidepressants are used for acute and maintenance treatment of major depressive disorder, but they also are used to treat panic disorder, agoraphobia, obsessive-compulsive disorder (OCD), social phobia, generalized anxiety disorder (GAD), posttraumatic stress disorder (PTSD), bulimia nervosa, and certain childhood disorders (e.g., enuresis, separation anxiety disorder). A comparison of commonly prescribed antidepressants is presented in Table 21–2.

Selective Serotonin Reuptake Inhibitors

The SSRIs are structurally dissimilar, but they share similar pharmacological properties involving selective serotonin reuptake inhibition. The SSRIs are remarkably versatile, and the following are FDA-approved indications:

- *Major depressive disorder*—citalopram, escitalopram, fluoxetine, paroxetine, and sertraline
- *OCD*—fluoxetine, fluvoxamine, paroxetine, and sertraline
- *Social anxiety disorder*—fluoxetine, paroxetine, and sertraline
- *Panic disorder*—paroxetine and sertraline
- *GAD*—escitalopram and paroxetine
- *PTSD*—paroxetine and sertraline
- *Premenstrual dysphoric disorder*—fluoxetine and sertraline
- *Bulimia nervosa*—fluoxetine

Metabolism

SSRIs are metabolized by the liver. Fluoxetine has the longest half-life, at 2–3 days, and its major metabolite, norfluoxetine, has a half-life of 4–16 days. Other SSRIs have half-lives ranging from 15 to 35 hours. All SSRIs are well absorbed, and peak plasma levels are reached within 4–8 hours.

Major Adverse Effects

SSRIs share a similar adverse-effect profile. Fluoxetine is the most likely, and escitalopram is the least likely, to induce adverse effects. Adverse effects are largely dose related and can include mild nausea, loose bowel movements, anxiety or hyperstimulation (leading to jitteriness, restlessness, muscle

TABLE 21–2. Commonly used antidepressants

Drug (trade name)	Sedation	Anti-cholinergic effects	Orthostatic hypotension	Sexual dysfunction	GI effects	Activation/ Insomnia	Half-life, hours	Target dosage, mg	Dosage range, mg/day
Selective serotonin reuptake inhibitors									
Citalopram (Celexa)	VL	None	None	VH	H	VL	35	20	10–60
Escitalopram (Lexapro)	VL	None	None	VH	H	VL	25	10	10–30
Fluoxetine (Prozac)	None	None	None	VH	H	VH	24–72	20	20–80
Fluvoxamine (Luvox)	M	None	None	VH	H	L	15	200	100–300
Paroxetine (Paxil)	L	L	None	VH	H	L	20	20	20–50
Sertraline (Zoloft)	VL	None	None	VH	VH	M	25	100	50–200
Other antidepressants									
Bupropion (Wellbutrin)	None	None	None	None	M	H	12	300	150–450
Desvenlafaxine (Pristiq)	L	None	VL	H	VH	M	10	50	50–400
Duloxetine (Cymbalta)	VL	L	None	VL	H	L	8–17	60	40–60

TABLE 21–2. Commonly used antidepressants *(continued)*

Drug (trade name)	Sedation	Anti-cholinergic effects	Orthostatic hypotension	Sexual dysfunction	GI effects	Activation/ Insomnia	Half-life, hours	Target dosage, mg	Dosage range, mg/day
Other antidepressants (continued)									
Levomilnacipran (Fetzima)	None	None	L	L	M	L	12	120	40–120
Mirtazapine (Remeron)	H	None	L	None	VL	None	20–40	30	15–45
Nefazodone (Serzone)[a]	H	None	L	None	M	VL	2–4	300	100–600
Trazodone (Desyrel)[a]	VH	VL	VH	None	M	L	6–11	400	300–800
Venlafaxine (Effexor)[a]	L	None	VL	H	VH	M	3–5	225	75–350
Vilazodone (Viibryd)	L	None	VL	VL	M	L	25	40	10–40
Vortioxetine (Trintellix)	VL	VL	VL	L	M	None	66	20	5–20
Tricyclics									
Amitriptyline (Elavil)[a]	VH	VH	VH	H	VL	None	9–46	150	50–300
Clomipramine (Anafranil)	VH	VH	VH	VH	VL	None	23–122	150	50–300

Somatic Treatments

TABLE 21–2. Commonly used antidepressants *(continued)*

Drug (trade name)	Sedation	Anti-cholinergic effects	Orthostatic hypotension	Sexual dysfunction	GI effects	Activation/ Insomnia	Half-life, hours	Target dosage, mg	Dosage range, mg/day
Tricyclics *(continued)*									
Desipramine (Norpramin)	M	M	M	H	VL	VL	12–28	150	50–300
Doxepin (Sinequan[a], Adapin[a])	VH	VH	VH	H	VL	None	8–25	200	50–300
Imipramine (Tofranil)	H	VH	VH	H	VL	None	6–28	200	50–300
Nortriptyline (Pamelor)	M	M	M	H	VL	None	18–56	100	20–150
Monoamine oxidase inhibitors									
Isocarboxazid (Marplan)	M	L	H	H	VL	L	—[b]	30	10–50
Phenelzine (Nardil)	L	M	VH	H	VL	L	—[b]	60	15–90
Tranylcypromine (Parnate)	None	M	VH	L	VL	M	—[b]	30–40	20–90

Note. GI=gastrointestinal; H=high; L=low; M=moderate; VH=very high; VL=very low.
[a]Brand no longer available in the United States.
[b]Maximum inhibition by monoamine oxidase inhibitors is achieved in 5–10 days.

tension, and insomnia), headache, insomnia, sedation, and increased sweating.

Sexual Dysfunction

SSRIs can decrease libido and cause ejaculatory delay or failure in men and anorgasmia in women. Management strategies include lowering the dosage, switching to one of the newer non-SSRI antidepressants (e.g., bupropion, duloxetine), or coadministering another medication as an antidote (e.g., bupropion, 75–300 mg/day). Sildenafil and other medications used to treat erectile disorder also are effective.

Hyperstimulation

Problematic hyperstimulation (fluoxetine is a major offender) can be managed by lowering the dosage, switching to another SSRI, or switching to one of the non-SSRI antidepressants. Propranolol (10–30 mg three times daily) can be helpful in treating subjective jitteriness and tremor. Benzodiazepines can be helpful as well.

Withdrawal Syndrome

When SSRIs are stopped, nausea and symptoms such as headache, vivid dreams, irritability, and dizziness can begin within days and continue for 2 weeks or longer. The exception is fluoxetine, which self-tapers because of its long half-life. Consider a slow drug taper to head off symptoms of withdrawal.

Serotonin Syndrome

Symptoms include lethargy, restlessness, confusion, flushing, diaphoresis, tremor, and myoclonic jerks. If untreated, serotonin syndrome can progress to hyperthermia, hypertonicity, rhabdomyolysis, renal failure, and death. Deaths have been reported in patients taking a combination of an SSRI and MAOI, presumably as a result of this syndrome; therefore, the drugs should never be coadministered.

Cytochrome P450

SSRIs inhibit one or more CYP isoenzymes to a substantial degree and have the potential to cause clinically important drug interactions. For that reason, take care when prescribing adjunctive or concurrent medication metabolized through this enzyme system. SSRIs can induce a several-fold increase in the levels of coprescribed drugs that are dependent on the inhibited isoenzymes for their clearance. Fluoxetine, fluvoxamine, and paroxetine are most likely to cause drug interactions, while citalopram and escitalopram have less potential to do so (Table 21–3).

FDA Warning

The FDA issued a warning in 2011 cautioning against prescribing citalopram at dosages greater than 40 mg/day because it could induce abnormal heart rhythms (through QT prolongation), including torsades de pointes.

Pregnancy/Lactation

All SSRIs are included in FDA risk Category C (risk to the fetus cannot be ruled out), except for paroxetine, which is in Category D (positive evidence of risk). The evidence base is largest with fluoxetine, which appears to be safe. SSRIs are secreted in breast milk.

Other Antidepressants

Bupropion

Bupropion has a unique chemical structure similar to those of psychostimulants. Bupropion is FDA-approved for treating major depression and smoking cessation. An extended-release formulation of the drug has been approved for seasonal affective disorder. Bupropion has been used off-label to treat attention-deficit/hyperactivity disorder.

Bupropion is rapidly absorbed, and peak concentrations are achieved within 2 hours. Elimination is biphasic, with an initial phase of approximately 1.5 hours and a second phase lasting approximately 14 hours. Bupropion is well tolerated with minimal effects on weight gain, cardiac conduction, or sexual functioning. Common adverse effects are headache, nausea, anxiety, tremors, insomnia, and increased sweating. Seizure risk appears to be dose-related and is particularly high at dosages >450 mg/day. Therefore, the drug is contraindicated in patients with a seizure disorder or an eating disorder that is associated with a lower seizure threshold.

TABLE 21–3. Selective serotonin reuptake inhibitors and newer antidepressants and potentially important drug interactions

Antidepressant	Enzyme system inhibited	Potential drug interactions
Fluoxetine	2D6	Secondary TCAs, haloperidol, type 1C antiarrhythmics
	2C	Phenytoin, diazepam
	3A4	Carbamazepine, alprazolam, terfenadine
Sertraline	2D6	Secondary TCAs, antipsychotics, type 1C antiarrhythmics
	2C	Tolbutamide, diazepam
	3A4	Carbamazepine
Paroxetine	2D6	Secondary TCAs, antipsychotics, type 1C antiarrhythmics, trazodone
Fluvoxamine	1A2	Theophylline, clozapine, haloperidol, amitriptyline, clomipramine, imipramine, duloxetine
	2C	Diazepam
	3A4	Carbamazepine, alprazolam, terfenadine, astemizole
Nefazodone	3A4	Alprazolam, triazolam, terfenadine, astemizole, carbamazepine
Duloxetine	1A2	Fluvoxamine, theophylline, clozapine, haloperidol, amitriptyline, clomipramine, imipramine
	2D6	Secondary TCAs, antipsychotics, type 1C antiarrhythmics, trazodone

Note. TCAs=tricyclic antidepressants.
Source. Adapted from Nemeroff CB, DeVane CL, Pollock BG: "Newer Antidepressants and the Cytochrome P450 System." *American Journal of Psychiatry* 153:311–320, 1996.

Duloxetine

Duloxetine is a potent inhibitor of serotonin and norepinephrine and is considered a selective serotonin-norepinephrine reuptake inhibitor (SNRI). The drug is FDA-approved to treat major depression, GAD, diabetic neuropathic pain, and fibromyalgia. Duloxetine is well absorbed and is metabolized in the liver mainly through CYP2D6 and CYP1A2. The half-life ranges from 8 to 17 hours. Duloxetine is well tolerated, with the most common adverse effects being insomnia, asthenia, nausea, dry mouth, and constipation. The drug is not associated with weight gain, and rates of sexual dysfunction are low. Duloxetine is metabolized through the CYP isoenzymes, creating a potential for drug interactions (see Table 21–3). Because of reports of hepatotoxicity, use the drug with caution in persons with chronic liver disease or in those with substantial alcohol use. Duloxetine should not be coadministered with an MAOI.

Levomilnacipran

Levomilnacipran is a newer SNRI with an FDA indication to treat major depression. The drug is well absorbed, has a half-life of about 12 hours, and is available in a slow-release formulation. Levomilnacipran is metabolized by the liver, mainly through CYP3A4. The drug and its metabolites are excreted renally. Common adverse effects include nausea, headache, dry mouth, and occasional increased blood pressure and pulse. Weight gain and rates of sexual dysfunction are low. Levomilnacipran should not be coadministered with an MAOI. Gradually reduce the dosage to avoid withdrawal symptoms.

Mirtazapine

Mirtazapine has a dual mode of action and enhances both serotonergic and noradrenergic neurotransmission but is not a reuptake inhibitor. Mirtazapine is FDA-indicated for treating major depression. The drug is well absorbed and is 85% protein-bound. It has a half-life of 20–40 hours. Mirtazapine is well tolerated but could cause somnolence, increased appetite, and weight gain. The drug has little effect on the cardiovascular system and minimally affects sexual functioning. Mirtazapine is unlikely to be associated with CYP-mediated drug interactions. One potential advantage is its early effect on reducing anxiety symptoms and sleep disturbance. Routine laboratory monitoring is not currently recommended because this adverse effect is rare. The drug is unlikely to be fatal in overdose. It should not be coadministered with an MAOI. Rare cases of agranulocytosis have been reported.

Trazodone

Trazodone is a weak inhibitor of serotonin but also blocks 5-HT$_2$ receptors. Trazodone has an FDA indication for treating major depression, but its main use has been in the off-label treatment of insomnia. The drug is readily absorbed orally, reaches peak plasma levels in 1–2 hours, and has a half-life of 6–11 hours. Trazodone is metabolized by the liver, and 75% of its metabolites are excreted in the urine. The drug should not be coadministered with MAOIs. Common adverse effects are sedation, orthostatic hypotension, dizziness, headache, nausea, and dry mouth. In rare cases, trazodone has been associated with priapism, which can be irreversible and require surgical intervention; warn men of this adverse effect.

Venlafaxine/Desvenlafaxine

Venlafaxine and its primary active metabolite, desvenlafaxine, are classified as SNRIs. Venlafaxine is indicated for treating major depression, but its extended-release formulation is FDA-approved for GAD, social anxiety disorder, and panic disorder. The drug is rapidly absorbed and is 98% bioavailable; its half-life is approximately 4 hours. Desvenlafaxine is available in a sustained-release formulation and is FDA-approved for treating major depression. Similar to the parent compound, desvenlafaxine is well absorbed and has a half-life of about 10 hours. Both venlafaxine and desvenlafaxine are metabolized by the liver and are excreted renally. Common adverse effects for both drugs are hyperstimulation, sexual dysfunction, and transient withdrawal symptoms. The drugs do not affect cardiac conduction or lower seizure threshold and generally are not associated with sedation or weight gain. Blood pressure monitoring is recommended with the use of either drug because of dose-dependent increases in mean diastolic blood pressure in some patients, particularly those with hypertension. The drugs are unlikely to inhibit CYP isoenzymes, and therefore drug–drug interactions are unlikely. Both drugs are contraindicated in patients taking MAOIs.

Vilazodone

Vilazodone is a serotonin reuptake inhibitor and 5-HT$_{1A}$ receptor partial agonist with little affinity for other serotonin receptors. Vilazodone is FDA-indicated for treating major depression. Drug concentrations peak 4–5 hours after administration, and absorption is increased when vilazodone is taken with food. Common adverse effects include nausea, diarrhea, headache, and somnolence. Vilazodone does not cause significant weight gain or sexual dysfunction. The drug should not be coadministered with an MAOI.

Vortioxetine

Vortioxetine inhibits the 5-HT transporter and has a variety of actions at five 5-HT receptor subtypes. It is FDA-approved for treating major depression. The drug is well absorbed orally, reaches peak plasma concentrations in 7–11 hours, and is 98% protein bound. The half-life of vortioxetine is about 66 hours, and steady-state concentrations are achieved after 2 weeks. The drug is metabolized through oxidation and subsequently by glucuronide conjugation. Nausea is a common side effect. The drug does not impact the cardiovascular system and does not alter the levels of other medications because it is not a hepatic enzyme inducer or inhibitor. Vortioxetine should not be coadministered with an MAOI. The drug should be tapered when discontinued.

Tricyclic Antidepressants

TCAs are believed to work by blocking the reuptake of both norepinephrine and serotonin at the presynaptic nerve ending. The tertiary amines (e.g., amitriptyline, imipramine, doxepin) primarily block serotonin reuptake, whereas the secondary amines (e.g., desipramine, nortriptyline, protriptyline) mainly block norepinephrine reuptake. Clomipramine is an exception because it is a relatively selective serotonin reuptake inhibitor. All of these drugs also block muscarinic, histaminic, and α-adrenergic receptors.

TCAs are well absorbed orally. They undergo an enterohepatic cycle, and peak plasma levels develop 2–4 hours after ingestion. They are highly bound to plasma and tissue proteins and are fat soluble. TCAs are metabolized by the liver, and metabolites are excreted through the kidneys. All TCAs have active metabolites, and there is as much as a 10-fold variation in steady-state plasma levels among individuals. Half-lives vary but generally are in the range of 1 day. Drugs that inhibit the CYP system, including chlorpromazine and other antipsychotics, disulfiram, cimetidine, estrogens, methylphenidate, and many SSRIs, tend to increase blood levels of TCAs.

Blood Levels

The established therapeutic range for imipramine (the total for imipramine plus its metabolite desipramine) is thought to be >200 ng/mL. Desipramine plasma levels >125 ng/mL are considered therapeutic. Optimal response for nortriptyline has been noted at 50–150 ng/mL. These therapeutic levels are based on steady-state concentrations, which are reached 5–7 days after administration of these medications. Blood should be drawn approximately 10–14 hours after the last dose of medication.

Adverse Effects

TCAs commonly cause sedation, orthostatic hypotension, and anticholinergic adverse effects such as constipation, urinary hesitancy, dry mouth, and visual blurring. Each TCA differs in its ability to cause these effects. Antihistaminic effects include sedation and weight gain. α-Adrenergic blockade causes orthostatic hypotension and reflex tachycardia. Carefully monitor blood pressure in geriatric patients because drug-induced hypotension can lead to falls and fractures. Other adverse effects of TCAs include tremors, pedal edema, myoclonus, restlessness or hyperstimulation, insomnia, nausea and vomiting, electroencephalographic changes, rashes or allergic reactions, confusion, and seizures. It is uncertain whether TCAs are teratogenic, but their use should be avoided in the first trimester of pregnancy. Cardiovascular side effects often are the most worrisome.

Cardiac Conduction

All TCAs prolong cardiac conduction, much as do quinidine or procainamide, and carry the risk of exacerbating existing conduction abnormalities. These medications should be used cautiously in patients with low-grade abnormalities such as first-degree atrioventricular block or right bundle branch block. Patients with a higher-grade block (e.g., second-degree atrioventricular block) should not take TCAs.

Withdrawal Syndrome

Patients who have been taking high dosages of TCAs for weeks or months could experience withdrawal syndrome. Symptoms begin within days after drug discontinuation and include anxiety, insomnia, headache, myalgia, chills, malaise, and nausea. This syndrome usually can be prevented with a gradual taper.

Monoamine Oxidase Inhibitors

MAOIs inhibit monoamine oxidase, an enzyme responsible for the degradation of tyramine, serotonin, dopamine, and norepinephrine. This action leads to an increase in central nervous system (CNS) levels of these monoamines. The four MAOIs available in the United States are isocarboxazid, phenelzine, tranylcypromine, and selegiline to treat major depression. A transdermal patch formulation of selegiline is also available. MAOIs are effective in treating panic disorder, agoraphobia, social phobia, PTSD, and bulimia nervosa. They also are thought to be particularly valuable for treating *atypical depression*.

MAOIs are readily absorbed orally. They do not have active metabolites and are renally excreted. MAOIs irreversibly inhibit monoamine oxidase, reaching maximum inhibition after 5–10 days. Plasma levels are not measured.

Adverse Effects

MAOIs have minimal anticholinergic and antihistaminic effects. They are potent α-adrenergic blockers, which results in a high frequency of orthostatic hypotension. Other common adverse effects include sedation or hyperstimulation (e.g., agitation), insomnia, dry mouth, weight gain, edema, and sexual dysfunction.

The most serious adverse effect results from the concomitant ingestion of an MAOI and substances containing tyramine, leading to severe hypertension and death or stroke in rare cases. Patients taking MAOIs must follow a special low-tyramine diet (Table 21–4). Because selegiline primarily affects monoamine oxidase B, there is no need to follow a tyramine-free diet with the 6-mg transdermal patch, but at higher dosages the diet is recommended. Patients taking MAOIs should avoid sympathomimetics, which could also produce a hypertensive crisis. MAOIs have a potentially lethal interaction with meperidine, the mechanism of which is not fully understood but might have to do with serotonin agonism.

When symptoms of a hypertensive crisis occur (e.g., headache, nausea, or vomiting), patients should immediately seek medical attention. Patients who do not have easy access to medical care should be advised to carry a 10-mg tablet of nifedipine (taken sublingually).

Use of Antidepressants

Begin treatment with an SSRI. Most patients will respond to a standard dosage, and frequent dosage adjustments are unnecessary. Patients with a history of cardiac conduction defects should receive an SSRI or a newer drug (e.g., bupropion, duloxetine, mirtazapine). Impulsive patients or those with suicidal ideation also should receive an SSRI or one of the newer agents because these agents are unlikely to be fatal in overdose. Nortriptyline, imipramine, and desipramine are the TCAs of choice because meaningful plasma levels can be measured.

For patients being treated for their first major depressive episode, continue the medication at the same dosage for at least 4–9 months after remission is achieved. When medication is tapered and discontinued, carefully monitor patients to ensure that their remission is stable. Consider chronic maintenance treatment to reduce the risk of relapse for patients with the following characteristics:

- Three or more lifetime major depressive episodes
- Double depression (i.e., major depression plus persistent depressive disorder)
- Two or more severe major depressive episodes in the past 5 years
- Depressive disorder complicated by comorbid substance use or anxiety disorder
- Age greater than 60 years at onset of major depressive disorder

TABLE 21–4. Dietary instructions for patients taking monoamine oxidase inhibitors

Foods to avoid

Cheese: all cheeses except cottage cheese, farmer cheese, and cream cheese

Meat and fish: caviar; liver; salami and sausage; smoked, dried, pickled, cured, or preserved meats and fish

Vegetables: overripe avocados, fava beans, sauerkraut

Fruits: overripe fruits, canned figs

Other foods: yeast extracts, fermented products, monosodium glutamate

Beverages: red wine, sherry, liquors

Foods to use in moderation

Chocolate

Coffee

Colas

Tea

Soy sauce

Beer, other wine

Medications to avoid

Over-the-counter pain medications except for plain aspirin, acetaminophen, and ibuprofen

Cold or allergy medications

Nasal decongestants and inhalers

Cough medications; plain guaifenesin elixir may be taken

Stimulants and diet pills

Sympathomimetic drugs

Meperidine

SSRIs, bupropion, desvenlafaxine, mirtazapine, nefazodone, trazodone, venlafaxine

Source. Adapted from Hyman SE, Arana GW: *Handbook of Psychiatric Drug Therapy.* Boston, MA, Little, Brown, 1987; Krishnan KRR: "Monoamine Oxidase Inhibitors," in *The American Psychiatric Publishing Textbook of Psychopharmacology,* 4th Edition. Edited by Schatzberg AF, Nemeroff CB. Washington, DC, American Psychiatric Publishing, 2009, pp. 389–401.

Medication trials generally should last 4–8 weeks. When the patient's symptoms do not respond after 4 weeks at the target dosage, increase the dosage or switch the patient to another antidepressant, preferably from a different class with a slightly different mechanism of action. When this regimen fails, nonresponders might benefit from the addition of lithium ("augmentation"). Response often is evident within a week with relatively low dosages (e.g., 300 mg three times daily). The SGAs aripiprazole and brexpiprazole both have FDA-approved indications as augmenting agents in adults with major depression. Other drugs that have been used for augmentation include pindolol, stimulants, and benzodiazepines. ECT is an option in patients whose depression does not respond to medication.

Rational Use of Antidepressants

1. Use SSRIs or one of the other newer antidepressants initially, and reserve TCAs and MAOIs for nonresponders.

2. Adjust dosages to fall within the recommended range, and each drug trial should last 4–8 weeks.

3. SSRIs generally are given once daily. TCAs can be administered as a single dose, usually at bedtime. MAOIs usually are prescribed twice daily but not at bedtime because they can cause insomnia. Bupropion is administered in two to three divided doses to minimize its risk of inducing seizures.

4. Although adverse effects appear within days of starting a drug, therapeutic effects might require 2–4 weeks to become apparent.

   • Monitor improvement by following target symptoms (e.g., mood, sleep, energy, appetite).

5. Patients with heart rhythm disturbances should be given one of the newer antidepressants that do not affect cardiac conduction (e.g., bupropion, mirtazapine, or an SSRI).

6. Antidepressants usually are unnecessary in patients with uncomplicated bereavement or adjustment disorders with depressed mood because these disorders are self-limiting.

Mood Stabilizers

Lithium, valproate, carbamazepine, and lamotrigine are used to treat bipolar disorder. In addition, all SGAs (except clozapine and lurasidone) have been FDA-approved to treat acute mania; two are indicated for maintenance treatment of bipolar disorder (aripiprazole, olanzapine); two are indicated for treating major depressive disorder associated with bipolar I disorder (lurasidone, quetiapine); and five are indicated for adjunctive treatment of acute mania in combination with lithium or valproate (aripiprazole, lurasidone, olanzapine, quetiapine, and risperidone). Additionally, quetiapine and a combined formulation of olanzapine and fluoxetine (Symbyax) are approved to treat the depressed phase of bipolar disorder. Commonly used mood stabilizers are listed in Table 21–5.

Lithium

Lithium carbonate, a naturally occurring salt, is a first-line treatment for bipolar mania and bipolar depression. It is one of the few drugs demonstrated to reduce suicide attempts and suicides. Lithium sometimes is used off label to treat aggression in patients with dementia, intellectual disability, or "acting out" personality disorders (especially borderline and antisocial types).

TABLE 21–5. Commonly used mood stabilizers

Drug (trade name)	Therapeutic plasma level	Dosage range, mg/day
Carbamazepine (Tegretol)	6–12 mg/L	400–2,400
Lamotrigine (Lamictal)	N/A	50–200
Lithium (Eskalith[a], Lithobid)	0.5–1.2 mEq/L	900–2,400
Valproate (Depakene, Depakote)	50–120 mg/L	500–3,000

[a]Brand no longer available in the United States.

Pharmacokinetics

Lithium is rapidly absorbed, and peak blood levels are obtained approximately 2 hours after ingestion. The elimination half-life is about 8–12 hours in manic patients and 18–36 hours in euthymic patients. (Manic patients who are overly active clear lithium from their system more rapidly.) Lithium is not protein bound and does not have metabolites. It is almost entirely excreted through the kidneys but can be found in all body fluids. Blood plasma levels are checked 12 hours after the last dose is given. Onset of therapeutic action often takes 5–7 days.

Dosing

The usual plasma level of lithium for treating acute mania is 0.5–1.2 mEq/L, but some patients do well outside this range. Maintenance dosages can be lower (0.5–0.7 mEq/L). In typical patients, lithium usually is started at 300 mg twice daily and then titrated until a therapeutic blood level is achieved. Dosage can be adjusted every 3–5 days. Check levels monthly for the first 3 months and every 3 months thereafter. Patients receiving chronic lithium therapy can be monitored less frequently. Lithium can be safely discontinued without a taper. It is available in liquid and extended-release formulations.

Adverse Effects

Thirst or polyuria, tremor, diarrhea, weight gain, and edema are relatively common side effects but tend to diminish with time.

Thyroid. Approximately 5%–15% of the patients undergoing long-term treatment develop clinical signs of hypothyroidism, which can be managed effectively with thyroid hormone replacement. Obtain baseline thyroid assays before starting lithium. Test thyroid function once or twice during the first 6 months of treatment and every 6–12 months thereafter as clinically indicated. Thyroid dysfunction reverses after lithium is discontinued.

Renal. Lithium is excreted through the kidneys and is reabsorbed in the proximal tubules with sodium and water. When the body has a sodium deficiency, the kidneys compensate by reabsorbing more sodium in the proximal tubules. Lithium is absorbed along with sodium and poses the risk of lithium toxicity with hyponatremia. Therefore, instruct patients to avoid becoming dehydrated from exercise, fever, or other causes of increased sweating. Avoid thiazide and other sodium-depleting diuretics because they may increase lithium levels. Nonsteroidal anti-inflammatory drugs have the potential to raise lithium levels and should be avoided.

Lithium could cause nephrogenic diabetes insipidus because lithium inhibits vasopressin, thereby reducing the ability of the kidneys to concentrate urine. As a result, many lithium-treated patients produce large volumes of dilute urine, which can be clinically significant for some individuals, particularly when output exceeds 4 L/day. Amiloride (e.g., 10–20 mg/day) or hydrochlorothiazide (e.g., 50 mg/day) can (paradoxically) reduce urine output. A nephrotic syndrome caused by glomerulonephritis occurs in rare cases and usually is reversible if lithium is discontinued.

Long-term lithium use has been associated with a decrease in the glomerular filtration rate, but significant decreases are uncommon. Reassess renal function every 2–3 months during the first 6 months of treatment and every 6–12 months thereafter as clinically indicated. If proteinuria or an increase in creatinine is evident, perform additional tests.

Metabolic. Long-term lithium treatment can lead to increased levels of calcium, ionized calcium, and parathyroid hormone. High levels of calcium can cause lethargy, ataxia, and dysphoria, symptoms that could be misattributed to depression rather than to hypercalcemia.

Cardiac. A reversible and benign flattening of the T wave on the electrocardiogram (ECG) occurs in 20%–30% of patients taking lithium. The drug could suppress the function of the sinus node and result in sinoatrial block. Thus, obtain an ECG before initiating lithium treatment in patients older than 40 years or in those with a history or symptoms of cardiac disease.

Dermatological.   Acne, follicular eruptions, and psoriasis have been known to occur in lithium-treated patients. Hair loss and thinning also have been reported. Except for cases of exacerbation of psoriasis, these reactions usually are benign.

Hematological.   Lithium induces a reversible leukocytosis, with white blood cell counts of 13,000–15,000/mm^3. The increase usually is in neutrophils and represents a step-up of the total body count rather than demargination.

Central nervous system.   Parkinsonian-like symptoms, such as cogwheeling, hypokinesis, and rigidity, could occur in lithium-treated patients. Cognitive effects, such as distractibility, poor memory, and confusion, also can develop with therapeutic levels of lithium.

Contraindications

Patients with a severe renal disease should not receive lithium. Lithium should be discontinued for at least 10–14 days after patients have had myocardial infarction. Lithium is contraindicated in the presence of myasthenia gravis because the drug blocks the release of acetylcholine. Because of the increased incidence of cardiovascular malformations in infants of mothers taking lithium (Ebstein's anomaly), the drug should be discontinued during the first trimester of pregnancy. Lithium is secreted in breast milk; therefore, mothers taking the drug should not breast-feed.

Valproate

Valproate is commonly used as an anticonvulsant and is FDA-approved for treating acute mania. An extended-release formulation is approved for both acute manic and mixed states. Valproate also is effective for long-term maintenance treatment of bipolar disorder.

Valproate is rapidly absorbed after oral ingestion, and its bioavailability is nearly complete. Peak concentrations occur in 1–4 hours; it is rapidly distributed and highly (90%) protein bound. The half-life of valproate is 8–17 hours. The drug is metabolized by the liver, primarily through glucuronide conjugation. Less than 3% is excreted unchanged. A plasma concentration of 50–125 μg/mL correlates with acute antimanic response. Valproate might be more effective than lithium in patients with mixed presentations, irritable mania, a high number of prior episodes of mania, or a history of nonresponse to lithium.

Common adverse effects include nausea, poor appetite, vomiting, diarrhea, tremor, sedation, and weight gain. Less frequent side effects include rashes, hematological abnormalities, and hair loss. Hepatic transaminase elevation can occur and is dose related but generally subsides spontaneously. A rare but fatal hepatotoxic reaction to valproate has been reported. The enteric-coated formulation of valproate generally is well tolerated and has a low incidence of gastrointestinal side effects. Neural tube defects have been reported with valproate use during the first trimester of pregnancy, and therefore, its use in pregnant women is not recommended.

Before starting valproate treatment, the patient should have a complete blood count and a liver enzyme measurement; the latter should be done periodically during the first 6 months and every 6 months thereafter. The drug is started at 250 mg three times daily, and the dosage can be increased by 250 mg every 3 days. Serum levels can be obtained after 3–4 days. Most patients will need 1,250–2,500 mg/day.

Carbamazepine

Carbamazepine, an anticonvulsant, is effective for treating acute mania and might be effective for maintenance treatment of bipolar disorder. The long-acting formulation of the drug is FDA-approved for treating acute manic or mixed episodes of bipolar disorder. Carbamazepine may be more effective in patients who cycle rapidly (i.e., more than four episodes per year) and who do not respond well to lithium. When carbamazepine is used to treat mania, there generally is a delay of 5–7 days before its effect is apparent.

Approximately 10%–15% of the patients taking carbamazepine develop a transient skin rash. Other common side effects include impaired coordination, drowsiness, dizziness, slurred speech, and ataxia. Many of these symptoms can be avoided by increasing the dosage slowly. A transient leukopenia causing as much as a 25% decrease in the white blood cell count occurs in 10% of patients. A smaller reduction in the white blood cell count may persist in some patients as long as they take the drug, but is not a reason for discontinuation. Aplastic anemia develops in rare cases.

Carbamazepine typically is started at a dosage of 200 mg twice daily and increased to three times daily after 3–5 days. Most patients will need 600–1,600 mg/day. The usual practice is to aim for anticonvulsant blood levels of 8–12 µg/mL, despite the fact that no dose-response curve has been established. Because carbamazepine induces CPY3A4, the drug may speed its own metabolism, and the blood level established at 3 weeks may be decreased by one-third at 6 weeks.

Before starting carbamazepine, the patient should have a complete blood count and an ECG. Warn the patient about the drug's rare hematological adverse effects. Investigate any indication of infection, anemia, or thrombocytopenia (e.g., petechiae), and obtain a complete blood count. Routine blood monitoring is unnecessary. Because carbamazepine is a vasopressin agonist, it can induce hyponatremia; therefore, convulsions or undue drowsiness should prompt obtaining serum electrolyte measurements. Carbamazepine has been linked with fetal malformations and should be avoided in pregnant women, especially during the first trimester. Breast-feeding is not recommended.

Lamotrigine

Lamotrigine, an anticonvulsant, is FDA-approved for the maintenance treatment of bipolar I disorder to delay the time to occurrence of mood episodes. The target dosage of lamotrigine is 200 mg/day, achieved through a slow titration (i.e., 25 mg/day for 2 weeks, 50 mg/day for 2 weeks, 100 mg/day for 1 week, then 200 mg/day). Slower titration is recommended for patients receiving valproate concomitantly with lamotrigine (e.g., lamotrigine 25 mg qod first 2 weeks). The oral bioavailability of the drug is 98%, and peak plasma concentrations occur initially at 1–3 hours, with a secondary peak at 4–6 hours. The drug is approximately 60% protein bound and is widely distributed in the body. Metabolism is through hepatic glucuronidation, and none of the metabolites are active. The half-life ranges from 25 to 35 hours.

Lamotrigine generally is well tolerated, and most adverse effects are minor. In rare cases, the drug can induce the potentially life-threatening Stevens-Johnson syndrome and toxic epidermal necrolysis. Instruct patients to discontinue the drug at the first sign of a rash. Rashes are more common among children. The drug is listed as Category C in terms of pregnancy risk, which indicates that harm to the fetus cannot be ruled out.

Rational Use of Mood Stabilizers

1. Use lithium, valproate, or carbamazepine initially for treating acute mania.

   • Monotherapy with SGAs, which are effective and well tolerated, is an excellent alternative.

   • The combination of lithium and valproate or a mood stabilizer with one of the SGAs might be effective when monotherapy fails.

2. A clinical trial of lithium, valproate, or carbamazepine should last 3 weeks; at that point, add or substitute another drug if there is minimal or inadequate response.

   • Drug nonresponders might respond to electroconvulsive therapy.

3. Lithium can be given as a single dose at bedtime when the dosage is less than 1,200 mg. Administer lithium with food to minimize gastric irritation.

4. Regularly monitor renal function and thyroid indices in patients treated with lithium. Monitor hepatic function in patients taking valproate.

5. Lamotrigine could be particularly helpful in preventing development of depressive episodes in patients with bipolar I disorder.

Anxiolytics

Anxiolytics are the most widely prescribed class of psychotropic drugs. They include barbiturates, nonbarbiturate sedative-hypnotics (e.g., meprobamate), benzodiazepines, and buspirone. Currently, only benzodiazepines and buspirone can be recommended because of their superior safety record.

Benzodiazepines

Benzodiazepines have a high therapeutic index, little toxicity, and relatively few drug–drug interactions. They are indicated for treating anxiety syndromes, sleep disturbances, musculo-skeletal disorders, seizure disorders, and alcohol withdrawal and for inducing anesthesia. Commonly used benzodiazepines are listed in Table 21–6.

Indications

Benzodiazepines are used for treating GAD, especially when severe. Many patients benefit when their anxiety is acute and problematic; these drugs generally should be given for short periods (e.g., weeks or months). Benzodiazepines have an antipanic effect, and both alprazolam and clonazepam are FDA-approved for treating panic disorder. Because of their abuse potential, they are considered second-line treatments.

Anxiety frequently complicates depression. Benzodiazepines often are coadministered with an antidepressant because they relieve anxiety symptoms quicker than antidepressants. When the antidepressant begins to take effect, the benzodiazepine can be withdrawn.

Benzodiazepines are effective for alleviating situational anxiety. DSM-5's *adjustment disorder with anxiety* is characterized by anxiety symptoms (e.g., tremors, palpitations) that occur in response to a stressful event. Adjustment disorders generally are brief, and for that reason, treatment with benzodiazepines should be time limited.

Benzodiazepines have established efficacy for short-term treatment of primary insomnia unrelated to identifiable medical or psychiatric illness. Their use as hypnotic agents is discussed in Chapter 12 ("Sleep-Wake Disorders").

Alcohol withdrawal syndromes commonly are treated with benzodiazepines because they are cross-tolerant with alcohol. Other uses of benzodiazepines include treating akathisia and catatonia and as an adjunct to pharmacotherapy for acute agitation and mania.

Pharmacokinetics

Benzodiazepines are rapidly absorbed and, except for lorazepam, are poorly absorbed intramuscularly. (Lorazepam is available for parenteral use.) Benzodiazepines are metabolized chiefly by hepatic oxidation and have active metabolites. Lorazepam, oxazepam, and temazepam are metabolized by glucuronide conjugation and have no active metabolites; they are relatively short acting and are the preferred benzodiazepines in geriatric patients.

TABLE 21–6. Benzodiazepines commonly used as anxiolytics

Drug (trade name)	Rate of onset	Half-life, hours	Long-acting metabolite	Equivalent dosage, mg	Dosage range, mg/day
Alprazolam (Xanax)	Fast	6–20	No	0.5	1–4
Chlordiazepoxide (Librium[a])	Fast	20–100	Yes	10.0	15–60
Clonazepam (Klonopin)	Moderate	30–40	No	0.25	1–6
Diazepam (Valium)	Very fast	30–100	Yes	5.0	5–40
Lorazepam (Ativan)	Fast	10–20	No	1.0	0.5–10
Oxazepam (Serax[a])	Slow	5–20	No	15.0	30–120

[a]Brand no longer available in the United States.

There are differences between single-dose and steady-state kinetics. Rapid-onset drugs tend to be lipophilic, a property that facilitates rapid crossing of the blood-brain barrier. Drugs with longer elimination half-lives accumulate more slowly and take longer to reach steady state. Washout of these drugs similarly is prolonged. Drugs with shorter half-lives reach steady state more rapidly but also have less total accumulation. Drugs with long half-lives tend to have active metabolites.

Adverse Effects

Benzodiazepines can cause drowsiness, somnolence, reduced motor coordination, and memory impairment, which could diminish with continued administration or dosage reduction. However, patients should be cautioned not to drive or use heavy machines, especially when starting these drugs.

Abuse Potential

All benzodiazepines have the potential for abuse and addiction. Benzodiazepines should be prescribed cautiously—if at all—in those with a history of substance use disorders and in patients with "acting out" personalities (e.g., borderline and antisocial personality disorders). When signs of dependence appear (e.g., drug-seeking behavior, escalating dosages), taper and discontinue the drug. Advise patients to avoid alcohol when taking benzodiazepines because the combination will cause greater CNS depression than will either drug alone.

Withdrawal

Discontinuation of benzodiazepines therapy after long-term treatment can lead to tremulousness, sweating, sensitivity to light and sound, insomnia, abdominal distress, and systolic hypertension. Serious withdrawal syndromes and seizures are relatively uncommon but are more likely with abrupt discontinuation. The effects of drug discontinuation can be minimized by gradually tapering the drug over 1–3 months. A slow taper is particularly important for benzodiazepines with short half-lives. When short-acting benzodiazepines are being discontinued, it may be helpful to switch the patient to a long-acting benzodiazepine before initiating a taper (e.g., from alprazolam to clonazepam).

Pregnancy/Lactation

Nearly all benzodiazepines fall into pregnancy risk Category D (positive evidence of fetal harm) or X (contraindicated in pregnancy), mainly on the basis of the occurrence of neonatal toxicity and withdrawal syndromes. For these reasons, avoid them during pregnancy and breast-feeding.

Buspirone

Buspirone is FDA-approved for the treatment of GAD. It does not produce sedation, nor does it interact with alcohol. There is no risk for abuse. Buspirone is ineffective for blocking panic attacks, relieving phobias, or diminishing obsessions or compulsions. Buspirone is well absorbed orally and is metabolized by the liver. Its half-life is 2–11 hours. Drowsiness, headache, and dizziness are common adverse effects. The usual dosage range is 20–30 mg/day in divided doses.

Rational Use of Anxiolytics

1. Benzodiazepines should be used only for limited periods (e.g., weeks to months) to avoid dependency, because most conditions they are used to treat are self-limiting.

   - Some patients will benefit from long-term benzodiazepine administration; in these situations, periodically assess patients for continuing need.

2. Benzodiazepines have similar clinical efficacy, so the choice of a specific agent depends on its half-life, the presence of metabolites, and the route of administration.

3. Once- or twice-daily dosing of the benzodiazepines is sufficient for most patients.

   - A dose given at bedtime might eliminate the need for a separate hypnotic.

   - Short-acting agents (e.g., alprazolam) are an exception to this recommendation because their dosing interval is determined by their half-lives.

4. Buspirone is not effective on an as-needed (prn) basis and is useful only for the treatment of GAD.

   - Because response to these agents takes several weeks, it is important to educate the patient not to expect quick results.

Agents for Extrapyramidal Side Effects

In treating any EPS, begin by reducing the dosage of the antipsychotic whenever possible or switching to an SGA with less potential to cause EPS. When these steps fail, consider using anticholinergics, amantadine, or propranolol as an adjunct.

Benztropine should be started at 1–2 mg/day, but geriatric patients should receive smaller dosages. The maximum allowable dosage is 6 mg/day of benztropine or its equivalent; delirium can occur at higher dosages. The adverse effects of anticholinergic medications—dry mouth, blurry vision, constipation, and urinary hesitancy—are additive with those of antipsychotics. Table 21–7 shows common agents used to treat EPS and their dosage ranges.

Intramuscular benztropine (1–2 mg) or diphenhydramine (25–50 mg) works within 20–30 minutes to alleviate acute dystonic reactions. Benztropine is the preferred agent because usually it does not cause sedation. Lorazepam (1–2 mg IM) also seems to work. Amantadine primarily is useful for treating symptoms of pseudoparkinsonism, such as tremors, rigidity, and hypokinesia. Treatment is initiated at 100 mg/day, and the dosage is increased to 200–300 mg/day. Onset of action occurs within 1 week. Adverse effects include orthostatic hypotension, livedo reticularis, ankle edema, gastrointestinal upset, and visual hallucinations in rare cases. Propranolol and other beta-blockers have been used to treat akathisia, which usually is not alleviated with an anticholinergic agent. Propranolol (e.g., 10–20 mg, 3–4 times daily) or another equivalent centrally acting beta-blocker works well.

Clonidine, an α_2-receptor agonist, also has been used for treating akathisia. The dosage of clonidine ranges from 0.2 to 0.8 mg/day given in divided doses. Orthostatic hypotension and sedation are the main adverse effects. Clonidine is a second-line agent after propranolol.

Electroconvulsive Therapy

ECT is a procedure in which a controlled electric current is passed through the scalp and selected parts of the brain to induce a grand mal seizure. Indications for ECT are listed in Table 21–8.

TABLE 21–7. Common agents used to treat extrapyramidal syndromes

Category	Drug (trade name)	Dosage range, mg/day	Comments
Anticholinergics	Benztropine (Cogentin)	0.5–6	Use 1–2 mg IM of benztropine or 25–50 mg IM of diphenhydramine for acute dystonia. Anticholinergics tend to work better at relieving the tremor of pseudoparkinsonism than hypokinesia.
	Diphenhydramine (Benadryl)	12.5–150	
	Trihexyphenidyl (Artane)[a]	1–15	
Dopamine facilitators	Amantadine (Symmetrel)[a]	100–300	Useful in situations in which anticholinergic adverse effects need to be avoided.
Beta-blockers	Propranolol (Inderal)	10–80	Works well for treating akathisia.
Alpha-agonists	Clonidine (Catapres)	0.2–0.8	Could cause orthostatic hypotension; therefore, increase dosage slowly. Works well for treating akathisia.

[a]Brand no longer available in the United States.

TABLE 21–8. Indications for electroconvulsive therapy

Medication-refractory depression

Suicidal depression

Depression accompanied by refusal to eat or take fluids

Depression during pregnancy

History of positive response to ECT

Catatonic syndromes

Acute forms of schizophrenia

Mania or schizoaffective disorder unresponsive to medication

Psychotic or melancholic depression unresponsive to medication

Relative contraindications to receiving ECT include recent myocardial infarction (i.e., within 1 month), unstable coronary artery disease, uncompensated congestive heart failure, uncontrolled hypertensive cardiovascular disease, and venous thrombosis. Space-occupying brain lesions and other causes of increased intra-cranial pressure, such as recent intracerebral hemorrhage, unstable aneurysms, or vascular malformations, are the only absolute contraindications to ECT. Psychotropic medications can be continued, although benzodiazepines should be reduced to the lowest possible dosage—or discontinued altogether—because they can interfere with induction of a seizure.

Patients are anesthetized with a short-acting anesthetic (e.g., methohexital, etomidate) and receive oxygen to prevent hypoxia, succinylcholine as a muscle relaxant to attenuate convulsions, and atropine or glycopyrrolate to reduce secretions and to prevent bradyarrhythmias. Glycopyrrolate does not cross the blood-brain barrier and might be associated with less postictal confusion than atropine in geriatric patients. After the patient is anesthetized, electrodes are placed on the scalp.

Bilateral electrode placement involves placing the electrode on each side of the head over the parietal lobes. With unilateral placement, one electrode is placed over the right temple and the other is placed at the vertex of the skull. Right unilateral placement is associated with less post-ECT confusion and memory loss.

A brief electrical stimulus is applied after placement of the electrodes. A bidirectional pulse wave is given rather than a continuous sinusoidal waveform because the pulse wave is associated with less cognitive impairment. Stimulation usually produces a 30- to 90-second tonic-clonic seizure. The seizure is accompanied by a period of bradycardia and a transient drop in blood pressure, followed by tachycardia and a rise in blood pressure. These physiological responses are attenuated by the pre-ECT medications. Patients usually receive 6–12 treatments at the rate of 2–3 times per week.

Adverse Effects

During ECT common adverse effects include brief episodes of hypotension or hypertension, bradyarrhythmias, and tachyarrhythmias; these effects rarely are serious. Fractures are uncommon now because of the use of muscle relaxants. Laryngospasm and prolonged apnea due to pseudo-cholinesterase deficiency, a rare genetic disorder, can occur. Seizures lasting longer than 2 minutes should be terminated (e.g., with intravenous lorazepam, 1–2 mg). Immediately after treatment, patients experience postictal confusion. Headache, nausea, and muscle pain also could be experienced after ECT. ECT can cause anterograde and retrograde amnesia that is most dense around the time of treatment. The anterograde component usually clears quickly, but the retrograde amnesia can extend back to months before treatment. All patients should be informed that permanent memory loss can occur.

Further Reading

DE Hert M, Schreurs V, Vancampfort D, VAN Winkel R: Metabolic syndrome in people with schizophrenia: a review. World Psychiatry 8(1):15–22, 2009

Jin H, Shih PAB, Golshan S, et al: Comparison of longer-term safety and effectiveness of 4 atypical antipsychotics in patients over age 40: a trial using equipoise-stratified randomization. J Clin Psychiatry 74(1):10–18, 2013

Kane JM, Fleischhacker WW, Hansen L, et al: Akathisia: an updated review focusing on second-generation antipsychotics. J Clin Psychiatry 70(5):627–643, 2009

Kane JM, Mackle M, Snow-Adami L, et al: A randomized placebo-controlled trial of asenapine for the prevention of relapse of schizophrenia after long-term treatment. J Clin Psychiatry 72(3):349–355, 2011

Krishnan KRR: Monoamine oxidase inhibitors, in The American Psychiatric Publishing Textbook of Psychopharmacology, 4th Edition. Edited by Schatzberg AF, Nemeroff CB. Washington, DC, American Psychiatric Publishing, 2009, pp 389–401

Lauriello J, Pallanti S (eds): Clinical Manual for the Treatment of Schizophrenia. Washington, DC, American Psychiatric Publishing, 2012

Leucht S, Komossa K, Rummel-Kluge C, et al: A meta-analysis of head-to-head comparisons of second-generation antipsychotics in the treatment of schizophrenia. Am J Psychiatry 166(2):152–163, 2009

Nemeroff CB, DeVane CL, Pollock BG: Newer antidepressants and the cytochrome P450 system. Am J Psychiatry 153(3):311–320, 1996

Perry PJ, Alexander B, Liskow BI, et al: Psychotropic Drug Handbook, 8th Edition. Baltimore, MD, Lippincott Williams & Wilkins, 2006

Rothschild AJ (ed): The Evidence-Based Guide to Antidepressant Medications. Washington, DC, American Psychiatric Publishing, 2012

Sackeim HA, Dillingham EM, Prudic J, et al: Effect of concomitant pharmacotherapy on electroconvulsive therapy outcomes: short-term efficacy and adverse effects. Arch Gen Psychiatry 66(7):729–737, 2009

Schatzberg AF, DeBattista C: Manual of Clinical Psychopharmacology, 8th Edition. Washington, DC, American Psychiatric Publishing, 2015

Schatzberg AF, Nemeroff CB: The American Psychiatric Association Publishing Textbook of Psychopharmacology, 5th Edition. Washington, DC, American Psychiatric Publishing, 2017

Vieta E, T'joen C, McQuade RD, et al: Efficacy of adjunctive aripiprazole to either valproate or lithium in bipolar mania patients partially nonresponsive to valproate/lithium monotherapy: a placebo-controlled study. Am J Psychiatry 165(10):1316–1325, 2008

Wisner KL, Bogen DL, Sit D, et al: Does fetal exposure to SSRIs or maternal depression impact infant growth? Am J Psychiatry 170(5):485–493, 2013

Index

Page numbers printed in **boldface** *type refer to tables, figures, or boxes.*

Benzodiazepines *(continued)*
    violent behavior and, 269
    withdrawal from, 226, 331,
        333
Benztropine, 306, 335
Bereavement. *See also* Grief
    adjustment disorders and,
        133
    antidepressants and, 323
    depressive symptoms and,
        88
Beta-blockers
    for panic disorder, 104
    for specific phobias or
        social anxiety
        disorder, 100
Binge-eating disorder, 160,
    161, 165, 166
Bipolar disorders. *See also*
    Mania
    in children and
        adolescents, 58
    diagnosis of, 77–81
    hypomania and, 80–81
    lamotrigine for, 329
    outcome of, 3
    psychotherapy for, 285
    rapid cycling and, 87
Bipolar type, of schizoaffec-
    tive disorder, 75
Bizarre content, of delusions,
    62
Bizarre or disorganized
    behavior, and psychotic
    symptoms, 23–24
Black box warning, for use of
    antidepressants by
    children and
    adolescents, 58
Blocking, and alogia, **27**
Blood plasma level, of
    antipsychotics, 304

Blood pressure monitoring,
    and venlafaxine, 317
Body clocks, and sleep cycles,
    180
Body dysmorphic disorder,
    116–117, 119
Body image, and anorexia
    nervosa, 160
Body mass index (BMI), and
    anorexia nervosa, 159
Body temperature, and
    circadian rhythm sleep-
    wake disorders, 180
Bone mineral densitometry,
    and eating disorders, 162
Borderline personality
    disorder (BPD)
    diagnosis of, **259–260**
    dissociative identity
        disorder and, 140
    group therapy for, 294, 298
    psychotherapy as first-line
        treatment for, 285
Boundary issues
    malpractice and, 281
    in treatment of personality
        disorders, 263
Brain imaging studies
    eating disorders and, 162
    obsessive-compulsive
        disorder and, 115
    posttraumatic stress
        disorder and, 128
    schizophrenia and, 70, 71
Brain injury
    major and mild neurocog-
        nitive disorders and,
        245–246
    memory impairment and,
        141
Breathing-related sleep
    disorders, 177–180

Dicyclomine, 225
Diet
    alcohol withdrawal and, 217
    eating disorders and, 164, 165
    monoamine oxidase inhibitors and, 321, **322**
Differential diagnosis
    of acute stress disorder, 131
    of adjustment disorders, 132–133
    of attention-deficit/ hyperactivity disorder, 53–54
    of autism spectrum disorder, 49–50
    of delusional disorder, 62
    of depersonalization/ derealization disorder, 142
    diagnostic process and, 6
    of dissociative amnesia, 140–141
    DSM system and facilitation of, 5
    of intellectual disability, 45
    initial interview and development of provisional, 18
    of mood disorders, 88
    of obsessive-compulsive disorder, 115
    of panic disorder, 103, **104**
    of phobic disorders, 100
    of posttraumatic stress disorder, 128
    of reactive attachment disorder, 124
    of schizoaffective disorder, 76

    of schizophrenia, 69–70, **71**
    of somatic symptom disorder, 148
    of violent and assaultive behaviors, 268
Diminished capacity, and insanity defense, 283
Diphenhydramine, 173, 306, 335
Disability, and legal issues, 278
Discontinuation, of benzodiazepines, 226–227. *See also* Tapering; Withdrawal
Disinhibited social engagement disorder (DSED), 123–124, 133
Disorganization dimension, of schizophrenia, 67, 68–69
Disorganized speech, and psychotic symptoms, 24, **25**
Disruptive, impulse-control, and conduct disorders
    clinical points for, 207
    compulsive shopping, 206
    conduct disorder, 203–205, 207
    intermittent explosive disorder, 201–203, 207
    Internet addiction, 206–207
    kleptomania, 205–206, 207
    oppositional defiant disorder, 199–201, 207
    pyromania, 205, 207
Disruptive mood dysregulation disorder (DMDD), 81–82

Family *(continued)*
    major and mild
        neurocognitive
        disorders and, 250
    mania and support or
        education for, 90
    violent behavior and
        removal of firearms
        from home, 270
Family history
    of phobic disorders, 99
    psychiatric interview and,
        13
Family therapy
    for alcohol use disorders,
        218, 220
    for conduct disorder, 207
    for eating disorders, 165, 167
    for posttraumatic stress
        disorder, 129
    for pyromania, 205
    for schizophrenia, 73,
        74–75
    techniques and uses of,
        296, 298
Fatigue, and major
    depressive episode, **82,**
    84
Fear, and separation anxiety
    disorder, **96.** *See also*
    Worry
Feeding and eating disorders
    avoidant/restrictive food
        intake disorder, 158
    clinical points for, 166–167
    pica, 157
    rumination disorder,
        157–158
Female orgasmic disorder,
    189
Female sexual interest/
    arousal disorder, 189

Fetal alcohol syndrome, 45,
    214
Fetishistic disorder, 196
Firearms
    suicide risk and, 271, 274
    violent behavior and, 270
Fixed dosing, of medication
    for alcohol use disorder,
    217, **218**
Flashbacks, and
    hallucinogen-related
    disorders, 222
Flattening or blunting, of
    affect, 15, 26–27
Flibanserin, and sexual
    dysfunctions, 192
Flight of ideas, 29–30
Flooding, and behavior
    therapy, 288
Flumazenil, 225
Fluphenazine, **302**
Fluoxetine
    adverse effects of, 309, **310,**
        313
    drug-drug interactions
        and, **315**
    eating disorders and, 165,
        166, 309
    intermittent explosive
        disorder and, 207
    obsessive-compulsive
        disorder and, 309
    oppositional defiant
        disorder and, 202
    panic disorder and, 104
    pediatric depression and,
        58
    pregnancy and, 314
    for specific phobias and
        social anxiety
        disorder, 100, 309
Flurazepam, **174**

Overdoses, of hallucinogens, 222

Overextending, and manic episode, 79

Overgeneralization, as cognitive distortion, **291**

Overvalued ideas, and delusions, 20

Oxazepam, **332**

Oxcarbazepine, 202, 207

Paliperidone, 76, **303**

PANDAS (pediatric autoimmune neuropsychiatric disorder associated with streptococcal infections), 57, 114

Panic attacks, 32, **101,** 102, 103

Panic disorder, 100–105, 309. *See also* Agoraphobia

Paranoid personality disorder, 256

Paraphilic disorders, 187, 195–198

Parasomnias, 181–183

Parental management training, and conduct disorder, 205

Parkinsonism, and neurocognitive disorder with Lewy bodies, 244. *See also* Pseudoparkinsonism

Parkinson's disease, and dementia, 247

Paroxetine
  adverse effects and dosages of, **310**
  drug-drug interactions and, **315**
  for generalized anxiety disorder, 107, 108, 309
  for major depressive disorder, 309
  for obsessive-compulsive disorder, 309
  for panic disorder, 104
  for posttraumatic stress disorder, 134
  pregnancy and, 314
  for specific phobias and social anxiety disorder, 100, 309

Partial hospitalization, for schizophrenia, 73, 74. *See also* Day care programs

Passivity, delusions of, 21–22

Pathological gambling, 230

Pathophysiology. *See* Etiology

Patient(s)
  abandonment of and malpractice suits, 281
  children as, 39
  delirium in elderly, 235
  management of violent, 268–269
  psychiatric interview and chance to ask questions, 19
  psychiatric interview and identification of, 11

Peabody Picture Vocabulary Test, **41**

Pediatric autoimmune neuropsychiatric disorder associated with streptococcal infections (PANDAS), 57, 114

Pedophilic disorder, 196

Pharmacotherapy *(continued)*
sexual dysfunctions
caused by, 190, **191**
for treatment of sexual
dysfunctions, 191,
192–193
Phencyclidine (PCP), 221, 222
Phenelzine, **312**
Phenylketonuria, 44
Phobias, and exposure
therapy, 288. *See also*
Specific phobia
Physical examination. *See also*
Medical conditions
assessment of children
and, 40–41
delirium and, 236
dissociative amnesia and,
141
eating disorders and, 162
major and mild neurocog-
nitive disorders and,
239, **240**
psychiatric interview and,
17–18
schizophrenia and, 70
substance use disorders
and, 211
Physicians, and somatic
symptom disorders, 149,
152. *See also* Doctor-
patient relationship;
Doctor shopping
Pica, 157
Pick's disease, 244
Pimavanserin, 247
Pimozide, 57, 63
Play, and assessment of
children, 39–40, 58–59
Polysomnographic studies,
and sleep-wake disorders,
170, 175, **176,** 179, 185

Positive reinforcement, and
behavior modification,
289
Positive symptoms, of
psychosis and
schizophrenia, 20, 66
Possible Alzheimer's disease,
242
Postnatal factors, in
intellectual disability,
45
Postpartum onset, of brief
psychotic disorder,
64
Posttraumatic stress disorder
(PTSD)
acute stress disorder and,
129
clinical management of,
128–129
clinical points for, 133–134
definition of, 125
differential diagnosis of,
128
DSM-5 diagnostic criteria
for, **125–127**
epidemiology of, 127
etiology of, 128
nightmares and, 129, 134,
183
selective serotonin
reuptake inhibitors
for, 309
subtypes of, 125
Posturing, and catatonic
motor behaviors, **26**
Poverty of speech, and
alogia, **27**
Prader-Willi syndrome,
117
Pramipexole, 184
Prazosin, 129, 134, 183

Vacuum pump device, and erectile disorder, 193, 194

Vaginismus, 189

Valbenazine, 306

Validity, of DSM system, 6

Valproate
adverse effects of, 328
antisocial personality disorder, 259
dosage range for, **325,** 328
mania and, 89, 327
pharmacokinetics of, 327–328
pregnancy and, 328
schizophrenia and, 73

Vardenafil, 193, 194

Varenicline, 229

Vascular neurocognitive disorder, and dementia, 245

Vegetative symptoms, of depression, 84

Venlafaxine
adverse effects of, **311,** 317
for anxiety disorders, 107, 108
dosage of, **311**
for posttraumatic stress disorder, 129
for specific phobias and social anxiety disorder, 100

Ventilatory insufficiency, and sleep-related hypoventilation, 179

Vilazodone, 318

Vindictiveness, and oppositional defiant disorder, **200**

Vineland Adaptive Behavior Scales, **41**

Violent and assaultive behaviors, as psychiatric emergencies
assessing risk for, 268, **269**
clinical points about, 270
etiology and pathophysiology of, 267–268
management of, 268–269

Visual hallucinations, 23, 67

Visuospatial ability, and mental status examination, 17

Vitamin E, and neurocognitive disorders, 249

Vocal inflections, lack of and affective flattening, 27

Vocalization, and rapid eye movement sleep behavior disorder, 183

Vocational rehabilitation, for schizophrenia, 74

Vortioxetine, **311,** 318

Voyeurism, and paraphilic disorders, 195, 196

Wechsler Intelligence Scale for Children—4th Edition (WISC-IV), **41**

Wechsler Preschool and Primary Scale of Intelligence (WPPSI), **41**

Weight changes
anorexia nervosa and, 159, 161
antipsychotics and, 307
depressive symptoms and, 31, **82,** 84
diabetes and, 153
eating disorders and, 162
sleep-related hypoventilation and, 180